Healthy Mom, Healthy Baby

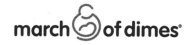
march of dimes®

Healthy Mom, Healthy Baby

The Ultimate Pregnancy Guide

Siobhan Dolan, M.D., M.P.H.,
and Alice Lesch Kelly

HarperOne
An Imprint of HarperCollins*Publishers*

HarperOne

HarperCollins books may be purchased for educational, business, or sales promotional use.
For information please e-mail the Special Markets Department at SPsales@harpercollins.com.

HarperCollins website: http://www.harpercollins.com

HarperCollins®, ®, and HarperOne™ are trademarks of HarperCollins Publishers.

FIRST EDITION

Designed by Terry McGrath

Library of Congress Cataloging-in-Publication Data
Dolan, Siobhan.
Healthy mom, healthy baby: the ultimate pregnancy guide /
Siobhan Dolan and Alice Lesch Kelly.
p. cm.
ISBN 978–0–06–211929–2
1. Pregnancy—Popular works. 2. Childbirth—Popular works.
3. Pregnant women—Health and hygiene—Popular works. I. Kelly, Alice Lesch. II. Title.
RG525.D645   2013

618.2—dc23   2012023458

13 14 15 16 17 RRD(C) 10 9 8 7 6 5 4 3 2 1

To Eilis, Niamh, and Liam, because I love you so much.
—SMD

To Steven and Scott, who will always be my babies.
—ALK

Contents

Notes to the Reader

Although this book contains the latest research-based pregnancy health information, the recommendations and advice contained in it should supplement, not replace, the instructions and advice of your health-care provider. You should see a qualified health-care provider for prenatal care. Decisions about your pregnancy should be made by you and your provider based on the specific circumstances of your health and your baby's health.

———

When we use the terms "health-care provider" or "provider," we are referring to a physician (doctor), physician assistant, nurse, nurse-practitioner, certified nurse-midwife, or any other licensed professional who provides prenatal care.

———

When we use the term "partner," we're talking about your spouse, your life partner, your baby's father, or any other person who gives physical and emotional support to you and your baby before, during, and after your pregnancy. We recognize that some readers have no partner; if that's the case for you, we hope you'll turn to friends and family members for support.

———

As you learn about pregnancy, you'll come across medical words that may be unfamiliar to you. We've included a glossary in the back of this book to help you with that.

Foreword

As a mom-to-be, you are looking ahead to the remarkable experience of pregnancy and the birth of your beautiful baby. Maybe you've been dreaming about having a child for some time. We at the March of Dimes have been thinking about babies for 75 years, and it's our mission to ensure a healthy birth for every baby. We're pleased to offer this wonderful new guide to support and empower your pregnancy, from preconception to birth.

Dr. Siobhan Dolan is your physician partner in this journey. We're proud to team up with her and Alice Lesch Kelly, an experienced health writer. Dr. Dolan is a mom herself. She's warm, friendly, thoughtful, and uniquely qualified with a combination of education and training as an obstetrician-gynecologist, geneticist, and public health specialist. Dr. Dolan has dedicated her career to finding ways to improve the health of mothers and babies and to prevent serious problems such as birth defects and premature birth.

Dr. Dolan recognizes that there's no one-size-fits-all approach to pregnancy care, because every woman has different life experiences, different circumstances and challenges. This may be your first child or you may have others. You may have a partner or be a single parent. You may or may not be working full-time. You may not be at your ideal weight or in perfect health. Dr. Dolan knows that despite these differences, what all moms-to-be have in common is that they want a healthy baby.

You may feel overwhelmed by the many changes and choices that a new baby brings into your life. Dr. Dolan answers the most common questions women ask and even those some women may be too embarrassed to raise. The book offers clear explanations for even the most complicated topics, providing practical tips, checklists, and basic steps for your own well-being and that of your new family. All of us at March of Dimes believe *Healthy Mom, Healthy Baby* is the best book to have by your side throughout your pregnancy.

The March of Dimes has been here to serve you since President Franklin D. Roosevelt founded our organization in 1938 in the quest for a vaccine against polio, an epidemic disease that once paralyzed or killed thousands of children every year. The March of Dimes has supported countless advances in newborn and child health: the nation's first newborn screening test, new treatments for heart defects and newborn jaundice, and the initiation of a regional system of neonatal intensive care units throughout the United States. More than four million babies are born each year in the United States. And the March of Dimes has helped each and every baby through research, education, vaccines, and breakthroughs.

So now you're having a baby of your own. Congratulations and all the best wishes for a very happy, healthy future!

Jennifer L. Howse, Ph.D.
President, March of Dimes
White Plains, New York

Acknowledgments

Writing this book was truly a collaborative effort. We thank everyone in the March of Dimes family who played a part in its conception, gestation, and delivery, especially:

Diane M. Ashton, M.D., M.P.H.
Lisa Bellsey
Wanda Beverly
Janis Biermann
Jennifer Coate
Todd Dezen
Alan Fleischman, M.D.
Lorraine Gore
David Horne
Jennifer L. Howse, Ph.D.
Michael Katz, M.D.
Chris Kehnle
Michele Kling

Alison Knowings
Karen Kroder
Christopher Lima
Elizabeth Lynch
Edward McCabe, M.D., Ph.D.
Richard Mulligan
Kieran O'Dowd
Motoko Oinuma
Chad Royal-Pascoe
Joe Leigh Simpson, M.D.
Doug Staples
Ann Umemoto
Frank Vitale

We also offer our sincere appreciation to our agent, Stephanie Tade; our editor, Gideon Weil; the HarperOne team—Laina Adler, Claudia Boutote, Mandy Chahal, Babette Dunkelgrun, Terri Leonard, Melinda Mullin, Suzanne Quist, Mark Tauber, and Michele Wetherbee; copy editor Kathy Reigstad; proofreader Judith Riotto; interior designer Terry McGrath; and Dr. Dolan's colleagues at the Albert Einstein College of Medicine/Montefiore Medical Center, Mary Alice Albert, Vincenc Aquilato, Nicole DeGroat, Catresa Johnson, Adrienne Kapel, Karla Damus, R.N., Ph.D., Susan Klugman, M.D., Robert Marion, M.D., and particularly Irwin R. Merkatz, M.D.

Finally, we thank our families, especially Dan Klein, Deirdre Dolan, and David A. Kelly.

Introduction

This book is about *you*.

You have the power to make smart choices that can have a major impact on your pregnancy and your baby's health. But in order to make the best choices, you need the most accurate, up-to-date pregnancy health information available. That's what you'll find in *Healthy Mom, Healthy Baby*.

This practical, easy-to-use book tells you exactly what you can do to have the healthiest pregnancy possible. Clear explanations, research-based recommendations, and sensible advice are here to inform and support you during every part of your journey to parenthood.

The following pages contain the information you need to make the healthiest choices before, during, and after pregnancy. When you face several options—for example, what kind of prenatal-care provider to see and whether to plan on using pain relief during delivery—we explain them in a way that helps you pick what's best for you. And when there is a single recommendation, we tell you what it is and why it's advised.

Healthy Mom, Healthy Baby also provides the information and support parents need if complications develop during pregnancy. Of course, most pregnancies turn out just fine. But in a small number of them, problems happen. For those women and their families we provide clear, current medical information and advice about how to achieve the best possible outcome for mom and baby.

We also tell you about the latest advances in pregnancy testing that can help you learn about your baby's health before birth. Genetic technology is developing rapidly. With the information in this book, you have the facts you need to make the best use of it.

START WHERE YOU ARE

Healthy Mom, Healthy Baby is for all women *at any stage of pregnancy.*

Ideally you're reading it before you get pregnant, when your lifestyle choices and medical decisions can have the greatest impact on your pregnancy and your baby's health.

But half of all pregnancies are unplanned, so there's a good chance that when you picked up this book you were already several weeks or months into your pregnancy.

That's okay. Learning about pregnancy health and taking steps to care for yourself and your baby can make a difference at *any* point in your pregnancy. Even if you're just a few weeks from giving birth, the choices you make from today on can increase your odds of having a safe birth and a healthy baby.

No matter what the situation, you can take meaningful, effective steps to improve your chances of having a comfortable pregnancy and a healthy, full-term baby.

Don't waste energy feeling upset with yourself if you missed opportunities before and during pregnancy to take care of your health. Focus on what you can do *now*. Start where you are, and commit to making healthy choices for the rest of your pregnancy.

Starting where you are includes your personal health. Sure, it's great to be in fantastic shape before you get pregnant—trim, fit, and perfectly healthy. But few of us begin pregnancy that way. You may be overweight or underweight. You may not eat many nutritious foods. You may smoke or have a sexually transmitted infection (STI). Perhaps you haven't seen a health-care provider in years and have a medical condition that's not under control. Whatever you do, don't throw up your hands and give up. Start where you are and get right down to taking care of yourself as best you can from now on.

No matter what the situation, you can take meaningful, effective steps to improve your chances of having a comfortable pregnancy and a healthy, full-term baby. Women who smoke can quit. Overweight women can improve their diet and start to exercise. Women with diabetes can get help with their blood sugar. Women who don't take prenatal multivitamins can start.

The focus is on what you *can* do, not what you *can't* do. And there's a lot you can do.

No book can guarantee a perfect pregnancy. Despite your very best efforts, complications can happen. But if they do, you still have power. The information and resources in *Healthy Mom, Healthy Baby* can help you get the best outcome possible and receive the support you need.

You have the power to take care of yourself and your baby. *Healthy Mom, Healthy Baby* shows you the way. The more you know, the healthier you—and your baby—will be.

A SOURCE OF TRUST

All of this information comes from a source you can trust. In the years since its founding in 1938, the March of Dimes has devoted $4 billion to supporting scientific research and educational initiatives that have improved the lives of moms and babies in the United States and throughout the world.

March of Dimes scientists helped eliminate polio, a disabling disease that had paralyzed countless children before the polio vaccine was introduced in the 1950s. They also promoted the use of a system called the Apgar score for evaluating a baby's health at birth. The score was created by Dr. Virginia Apgar, who worked tirelessly with the March of Dimes to advance the cause of prenatal health. Since its inception, the Apgar score has been used to assess the health of billions of babies worldwide.

The March of Dimes has led the effort to spread the word about the importance of folic acid supplements for women of childbearing age and helped bring about folic acid fortification of the grain and cereal supply. Since folic acid fortification began, the United States has seen a 26 per-

> The March of Dimes has devoted $4 billion to supporting scientific research and educational initiatives that have improved the lives of moms and babies in the United States and throughout the world.

cent decrease in defects of the neural tube, which eventually develops into a baby's brain and spine.

Scientists funded by the March of Dimes are also hard at work in the fields of genetics, high-risk pregnancy, and advanced care of critically ill newborns.

Most recently, the March of Dimes has committed millions of dollars to researching the causes of preterm birth and educating women and health-care providers on how to prevent it. Since the start of this initiative, preterm birth rates in the United States have gone down by 5 percent. Research is under way to find ways to lower preterm birth rates even more.

The March of Dimes is working toward a future when all children are born healthy. *Healthy Mom, Healthy Baby* helps bring us all closer to reaching that goal.

HOW TO USE THIS BOOK

Healthy Mom, Healthy Baby is packed with information. But we don't want you to feel overwhelmed—you have enough on your mind without having to wade through a medical encyclopedia. That's why we've organized this book in a way that makes it clear and easy to use.

Each chapter focuses on one topic. Within the chapter we include information that pregnant women need to have. For some topics, we include additional information in the "In Depth" section in the back of the book. This chapter structure makes it easy for you to skip subjects that don't relate to you and focus on precisely what you need and want to know.

Go online: The March of Dimes has information-packed websites (marchofdimes.com in English, and nacersano.org in Spanish) that feature articles and videos, online support groups, and places to connect with other parents and share your stories.

We also share many resources available from the March of Dimes, including information-packed websites (marchofdimes.com in English, and nacersano.org in Spanish) featuring articles and videos, online support groups, and places to connect with other parents and share your stories.

Healthy Mom, Healthy Baby gives you all the information you need to make sure you have the happiest, healthiest, safest pregnancy possible.

Chapter One

The Journey Begins

Congratulations—you're pregnant!

Pregnancy is an amazing journey. Your body undergoes incredible changes as your baby grows and develops inside you. Before you know it, you'll hold a beautiful newborn in your arms.

Your body knows exactly how to build a baby. You don't have to tell your body when to make a placenta or how to manufacture the extra blood needed to carry oxygen and nutrients to your baby. In some ways, you're just an observer, watching as your body uses its natural wisdom to bring a new person to life.

But that doesn't mean you can't help your body do its best to grow the healthiest baby possible. There are so many ways to support your body as it works to bring your child to life.

Understanding what your body and your baby need during pregnancy allows you to make smart choices. Just making the decision to take a prenatal multivitamin every day, or to shield yourself from unsafe chemicals in your environment, can have a huge impact in protecting your baby's health.

No matter where you are in your pregnancy, you have a wonderful opportunity to boost your chances of having a problem-free pregnancy and a healthy baby. You can begin making a difference right away.

By deciding to take charge of your health, you're taking a leap toward a healthy, happy future for yourself and your baby.

PRENATAL CARE MATTERS

Getting good medical care during pregnancy is the greatest gift you can give your baby and yourself. The care you receive while you're pregnant—called prenatal care—can help you and your baby be as healthy as possible.

Prenatal care is more than just checkups and tests. It also includes education about pregnancy and childbirth, information about how to prevent problems, guidance on ways to improve health behaviors, and advice on making the healthiest choices for you and your baby.

During prenatal-care visits, your health-care provider checks on your pregnancy and your baby's development. Should problems come up, your provider can spot them early, often when they're easiest to treat.

> *One of the most effective steps toward a healthy pregnancy is taking daily prenatal multivitamins with 600 to 800 micrograms of folic acid, a nutrient that helps prevent neural tube defects—birth defects of the brain and spine. If you haven't been taking multivitamins, pick some up from your local drugstore and start today.*

Good prenatal care is crucial for all women, but it's especially important if you have medical conditions such as diabetes, high blood pressure, seizure disorder, or other problems that can interfere with a healthy pregnancy. Even if you've already had a baby, and even if you're starting your pregnancy in excellent health, prenatal care matters.

Start getting prenatal care as early in your pregnancy as possible. Ideally you should see a prenatal-care provider shortly after you conceive—the earlier you start receiving pregnancy care, the better. But even if several months into your pregnancy you haven't seen a provider yet, you can still benefit from prenatal care.

PICKING YOUR PROVIDER

Deciding what kind of prenatal health-care provider to see is one of the first health decisions you make during pregnancy. You can choose to see a doctor, a nurse, or a certified nurse-midwife—or a combination of providers on a team that might also include a physician assistant. How do you decide? The answer is different for everyone. Choose the provider you think is best. If your health needs suggest that you should be seeing a different kind of provider, the person you see will refer you to someone else. What matters most is that you're getting the prenatal care that's right for you.

Obstetrician-gynecologists (OB-GYNs) OB-GYNs are medical doctors who specialize in women's health and take care of women during pregnancy, labor, and childbirth. OB-GYNs can deliver babies vaginally or, if necessary, surgically with a cesarean section (c-section). In addition to completing medical school, OB-GYNs do four years of residency training and must pass a test administered by the American Board of Obstetrics and Gynecology to become board-certified. Roughly 80 percent of women see an OB-GYN.

Planning ahead? If you aren't pregnant yet, call your provider for a preconception checkup. See "Preconception: Preparing for a Healthy Pregnancy" (page 213) to learn all about preconception care.

Maternal-fetal medicine specialists (MFMs) Also known as perinatologists, MFMs care for women having high-risk pregnancies. MFMs are obstetricians who complete three additional years of training after medical school in the area of pregnancy and fetal complications.

Family physicians These are medical doctors who care for all members of the family, from babies to the elderly. Many (but not all) family physicians offer pregnancy care and childbirth services.

Nurse-practitioners (NPs) NPs are registered nurses who receive additional training in a specialty area such as women's health, pediatrics, or family health. NPs work in a variety of settings, including hospitals, community clinics, doctors' offices, and walk-in clinics. They typically work as part of a team of providers that includes medical doctors, specialists, and midwives. NPs may provide prenatal care but they do not deliver babies unless they are also certified nurse-midwives.

Physician assistants (PAs) PAs receive extensive medical training and must pass a national certification exam in order to practice medicine as part of a team (along with medical doctors) in hospitals, clinics, and other settings. PAs can deliver babies if they are trained and certified in obstetrics.

Certified nurse-midwives (CNMs) CNMs are registered nurses who are specially trained to care for women and their babies during pregnancy, labor, and birth, as well as after birth, and who are certified by the American Midwifery Certification Board. CNMs attend almost 8 percent of births in the United States, mostly in hospitals and birthing centers.

CNMs typically provide prenatal care and deliver babies of healthy women whose pregnancies are considered low-risk. CNMs generally do not manage high-risk pregnancies and do not perform surgical procedures such as c-sections, but they may work with obstetricians on high-risk cases.

Midwives who are not CNMs are known as lay midwives. Regulation and licensing of lay midwives varies by state; in some states, uncertified midwifery is illegal. The March of Dimes advises against using lay midwives.

With all these options, making a choice can be difficult. If you aren't sure which provider to see for your prenatal care, ask for recommendations from your primary-care provider, trusted friends, and family members. The ideal provider is not just medically qualified, but someone whom you respect, who respects you, and who is willing to offer support and answer all of your questions.

The provider you choose will be with you during one of the most important experiences of your life, so you want to pick someone you feel good about. After all, you're going to be spending a lot of time together!

Q: *How long does pregnancy last?*

A: *The length of a full-term pregnancy is described in several ways:*

- *__Forty weeks from the first day of your last period.__ This is the standard way that providers date a pregnancy during prenatal care.*

- *__Three trimesters.__ The first trimester is weeks 0–13; second trimester, weeks 14–27; third trimester, weeks 28–40.*

- *__Nine months.__ Most people think of pregnancy as lasting nine months, but nine calendar months is only about 36 or 37 weeks. A full-term pregnancy is 39 to 41 weeks, with your due date at 40 weeks, so pregnancy actually lasts closer to 10 months.*

Your provider should also be someone who can deliver your baby in the hospital or birthing center you choose and whose office location and hours fit your schedule.

Another consideration is whether the provider works alone or in a group. If it's a group practice, ask questions about their policies. Will you see one provider throughout your pregnancy, or whichever provider is on duty at the time of your appointment? Who will attend your birth if your chosen provider is off duty or away on vacation? Some women don't care which provider they get; others prefer having one person see them throughout their pregnancy.

Be sure your provider accepts your health insurance. For coverage details, check with your insurance carrier and the provider's business office. Find out about deductibles, copays, allowable tests and procedures, and whether/when you need preapprovals or referrals. Understanding the fine print in your health insurance policy now can help prevent expensive surprises later.

Finally, find a provider you like and feel comfortable with. There is no *one* perfect provider. Think of all of these considerations, and choose the provider who is right for you.

IN DEPTH

Prenatal Care for Women Without Health Insurance

See page 240

YOUR FIRST PRENATAL VISIT

Your first prenatal visit can be overwhelming. There's so much to talk about with your provider—so many questions to ask and answer. You can help the visit go smoothly and quickly by gathering whatever information you can put your hands on before your appointment and taking it with you.

For example, make note of the names and amounts of any medications you take, the dates of your vaccinations, details about your family health history, and the timing of your most recent menstrual period.

During your first prenatal appointment, your provider will determine your due date, also known as your estimated date of delivery (EDD). Although most women don't give birth on their actual due date, providers use the date to monitor a pregnancy and a baby's growth and to determine when to give certain tests.

Your due date is calculated using the date of the first day of your most recent menstrual period. Even though most women conceive about two weeks after the first day of menstruation, those two weeks are included in the count of a full-term 40-week pregnancy. Don't worry if your cycles are irregular—your provider will probably do an ultrasound early in your pregnancy to verify your due date.

You can calculate your due date using this online pregnancy tool: marchofdimes.com/pregnancy/ yourbody_duedate.html.

Here's an easy way to calculate your due date: Start with the first day of your most recent period. Add seven days, then count backward three months.

Say the first day of your most recent period was February 12. Add seven days (February 19) and then count back three months (November). Using this formula, your due date would be November 19.

Here are some other things you can expect during your first appointment with your prenatal-care provider:

A full physical exam This includes a check of your height, weight, blood pressure, heart, lungs, and breasts.

A pelvic exam Nobody likes pelvic exams, but they're an important way for your provider to check the health of the parts of your body that are hard at work building your baby.

This exam has two parts: the speculum exam and an internal exam. During the speculum exam, your provider gently places an instrument called a speculum into your vagina to open it up for visual inspection of the vagina and cervix, to collect cells from your cervix for a Pap smear, and to test for STIs, including gonorrhea, chlamydia, and human papillomavirus.

Once the speculum is removed, your provider performs the internal pelvic exam by inserting the gloved fingers of one hand into the vagina to feel the cervix, and placing the other hand on your belly to feel the uterus and ovaries between the two hands.

Usually the internal exam also includes a rectal exam, during which your provider inserts one gloved finger in the vagina and one in the rectum to feel for irregularities in the rectum, cervix, uterus, and ovaries. Fortunately, this part of the checkup is over before you know it.

A conversation about multivitamins One of the best things you can do for your baby is also one of the easiest: take a daily multivitamin pill. That one little pill can have a big impact on your baby's health.

A prenatal multivitamin is packed with the vitamins and minerals you and your baby need during pregnancy. They're all helpful, but perhaps the most important vitamin early in pregnancy is folic acid. A kind of B vitamin, folic acid helps lower a baby's risk of having a defect in the neural tube, the structure that eventually develops into the brain and spine.

Folic acid is powerful. If all women of childbearing age were to get the recommended amount of folic acid from the foods they eat or from vitamin supplements before they got pregnant and during the first months of pregnancy, up to 70 percent of neural tube defects could be prevented.

> Women say the number one reason they don't always take their prenatal multivitamin every day is that they forget. To be sure you remember, take it at the same time every day—right before bed or after you brush your teeth in the morning. Before you know it, taking your multivitamin will become a habit.

Ideally you were taking daily multivitamins containing the recommended preconception dose of 400 micrograms of folic acid before you conceived. Once you get pregnant, your recommended dose of folic acid goes up to 600 to 800 micrograms.

Your provider may recommend taking larger amounts of folic acid if you have certain risk factors. For example, women with neural tube–related problems during previous pregnancies, or with medical conditions such as diabetes, epilepsy, or sickle cell disease, may be advised to take as much as 4,000 micrograms (equal to 4 milligrams) of folic acid each day. But don't take high doses of folic acid or any other supplement unless told to do so by your provider.

Prenatal vitamins are easy to get. They're available over the counter or by prescription. Their vitamin and mineral content can vary, so check with your provider to decide which is best for you. Keep in mind that when it comes to multivitamins, taking too much can be unsafe. For example, excess vitamin A can harm your liver and raise your baby's risk of birth defects. So stick with the amount your provider recommends.

A discussion about medications Think of this as a quick check of your medicine chest. Your provider wants to know about any prescription or over-the-counter drugs you take, as well as any supplements and herbs. Some medications can raise the risk of birth defects and other problems in a developing baby, so it's important not to take them during pregnancy. If any of your medications pose a potential danger, your provider will advise you about stopping them and, if necessary, switching to safer ones. Many medications that are not recommended during pregnancy can be replaced with low-risk alternatives.

IN DEPTH

Drug Safety During Pregnancy

See page 242

Questions about your health and pregnancy history Your provider will want to know details about past and current health issues, along with information about previous pregnancies, because they may affect your pregnancy health. It's especially important to tell your provider if you've ever had preterm labor or a preterm birth.

Q: *Can I use herbal products while I'm pregnant?*

A: *It's best to stay away from them, or to use them only with the approval of your prenatal-care provider. Many of these products have not been tested or regulated, and they may contain varying amounts of ingredients or substances that are unsafe for an unborn baby.*

Questions about your family's health and genetic history Having details about medical and genetic problems in your family and your baby's father's family helps your provider know more about what health issues to look out for. Your provider can tell you about the risk of having a baby with certain genetic conditions, some of which increase in likelihood with maternal age. If you or your provider has concerns, you may be referred to a genetic counselor who can help you understand your risks and explain your testing options. Some providers refer all patients to a genetic counselor. For more about genetic screening during pregnancy, see chapter 9.

A plan for managing medical problems If you have any known medical conditions, such as diabetes, thyroid disease, or other health problems, talk with your provider about them. Women with medical conditions are sometimes advised to get their prenatal care from a maternal-fetal medicine doctor who cares for women with high-risk pregnancies. Appointments with a doctor who specializes in treating certain conditions may also be recommended. Women with medical conditions can usually have perfectly healthy babies—but they must get the care they need from appropriate providers.

A urine test The contents of your urine can tell your provider some important facts about your health. In this simple test, you give a small urine sample in a cup. The sample is tested for several things, including sugar (a sign of diabetes), protein (a sign of kidney problems), and bacteria (a sign of infection in the urinary tract).

Blood tests Many women can't believe how many tubes of blood are taken at the first prenatal visit, but there's a lot to check. Your blood provides a wealth of information, including:

- **Blood type.** This establishes the basic A, B, O, or AB type.

- **Rh factor.** Rh factor is an inherited protein found on the surface of red blood cells. Most people have this protein and are called Rh-positive; those people who don't have it are called Rh-negative. Rh-negative women with Rh-positive partners are at risk of having a baby with a form of anemia called Rh disease, which can cause fetal brain damage, heart failure, or death. Fortunately, Rh disease can usually be prevented with injections of a blood product known as Rh immune globulin (commonly known as RhoGAM) at 28 weeks of pregnancy and again after birth. RhoGAM is also given to Rh-negative women at the time of miscarriage or amniocentesis, when they might be exposed to fetal blood cells. This helps prevent the woman's body from mounting a harmful immune response during a future pregnancy.

- **Red blood cell count, or hematocrit.** Having enough red blood cells is important during pregnancy, because these cells pick up oxygen in your lungs and carry it throughout your body. Having too few red blood cells is called anemia, a condition that affects about half of women at some time during their pregnancy. Left untreated, anemia can contribute to preterm birth and low birthweight, but it is usually easily treated with iron supplements. Prenatal multivitamins typically contain the amount of iron recommended during pregnancy (27 milligrams), but women with anemia may need extra.

- **Glucose level.** If you have extra glucose (sugar) in your blood, it could be a sign that you have diabetes, a disease in which your body doesn't use sugar properly. If your glucose level is high, you can have further tests to check for diabetes.

- **Infection.** Blood tests check for STIs such as HIV, syphilis, and hepatitis B. Your provider may choose to test you for a nonsexually transmitted infection such as toxoplasmosis as well.

- **Rubella immunity.** You probably got a vaccine for rubella (also known as German measles) during childhood. However, rubella immunity doesn't always last into adulthood. A blood test checks on rubella immunity by measuring rubella antibodies in your blood. It's important to know whether you're immune, because if you're not and you are exposed to German measles during pregnancy, your baby could be at risk of developing birth defects. Usually the rubella vaccine isn't recommended for pregnant women—it's best to get it before you become pregnant. If you're not immune, you can take extra care not to expose yourself to anyone with rubella while you're pregnant.

- **Varicella immunity.** This checks to see whether you are immune to chickenpox, either because you had the disease yourself or you received the vaccine. If you are not immune, it is best to avoid contact with anyone who has chickenpox while you're pregnant.

- **Thyroid hormone level.** Your provider may opt to check the thyroid hormone levels in your blood. The thyroid, a butterfly-shaped organ in your neck, produces hormones that help regulate many body functions. If the thyroid is not working right, it can produce too much or too little thyroid hormone, either of which can be harmful to a baby. If tests show hyperthyroidism (an overactive thyroid) or hypothyroidism (an underactive thyroid), the condition can be treated with surgery or medications that are safe during pregnancy. Some medical experts believe every pregnant woman should receive a thyroid blood test.

A flu shot Nobody likes shots. But if it's flu season (October through May), it really is important to get a flu shot. The flu can cause more trouble in pregnant women than in other adults. Flu-related complications can be much worse for pregnant women, and having the illness can increase your baby's chance of being born early. Getting a flu shot helps your baby after birth, too. Babies born to moms who got their flu shot during pregnancy are less likely to get sick with flu early in life. That's a lot of benefit from one quick shot. Flu shots are considered safe for pregnant women.

An appointment for a first-trimester ultrasound Think of this as a date for your baby's first photograph—and an exciting chance to "see" your baby for the very first time. Many providers recommend that their patients have a first-trimester ultrasound (sometimes called a sonogram) between the 11th and 13th weeks of pregnancy.

During an ultrasound, your provider (or an ultrasound technician) inserts a device called a transducer into your vagina; the transducer sends out sound waves that create pictures of your baby on a computer screen. The test has no known risks to you or your baby. A first-trimester ultrasound is used to confirm your due date and check for signs of problems in your baby. It can also show whether you are carrying more than one baby.

A discussion about prenatal screening tests While you're pregnant, you have the choice of receiving screening tests that look for signs of possible health or genetic problems in your baby. Some are offered to every woman; others are used mainly in women with certain risk factors. If screening tests show an elevated risk of any problems, further testing (called diagnostic testing) may be performed. Prenatal testing is explored in detail in chapter 9.

Answers to your questions about the safety of workplace chemicals Most workplaces are pretty safe, but some expose workers to chemicals that are risky during pregnancy. If you work with chemicals, your provider can help you determine what precautions you should take and whether it's safe for you to keep working with them during pregnancy. For more on environmental safety, see chapter 8.

THE IMPORTANCE OF GOOD LIFESTYLE CHOICES

No one likes to admit when she is doing something she shouldn't be. But it's important to tell your provider if you're smoking, drinking, or using drugs. These habits affect the kind of prenatal care you should receive. Your provider needs to know about them in order to help you have the healthiest pregnancy possible.

Don't let shame or embarrassment prevent you from being 100 percent truthful about your lifestyle choices. And don't worry about being judged. Your provider will support you, offering information and encouragement to help you quit. Pregnancy is a time when many women who have tried and failed in the past finally find the motivation to quit.

Don't let shame or embarrassment prevent you from being 100 percent truthful with your provider about your lifestyle choices.

And while this may be hard, if you smoke, drink, or use drugs, try to stop. Even if you've already been pregnant for several months, quitting now makes a big difference. Don't waste energy on guilt or self-blame. Focus on doing what you can to quit. Breaking those bad habits will make your life and your baby's life healthier and happier.

Smoking Moms who smoke during pregnancy have a higher risk of complications such as stillbirth. In addition, their babies are more likely to be born too small and too early.

Even secondhand smoke can contribute to sudden infant death syndrome, ear infections, and a range of breathing problems, such as asthma, in babies. So ask everyone who lives with you to quit smoking today, and start getting your home ready for your new baby. It's *never* too late to stop smoking. Quitting smoking *today* can improve your baby's chances of being born healthy.

IN DEPTH

If You Need Help Quitting

See page 243

Drinking It may seem like a single drink or two now and then can't be that bad, but it really is important to stay away from alcohol during pregnancy. If a mom drinks, her baby drinks: alcohol passes through the placenta and directly into the baby's blood, brain, and other organs. A baby's body breaks down alcohol much more slowly than an adult's, so alcohol remains in a baby's body far longer than it does in an adult's.

Alcohol can cause miscarriage, preterm birth, stillbirth, and a range of physical and mental birth defects, including intellectual disability, learning difficulties, emotional and behavioral problems, an abnormally formed brain, and structural changes to the heart, face, and organs. The term "fetal alcohol spectrum disorders" (FASDs) is used to describe the many problems associated with exposure to alcohol before birth. The babies of women who binge drink or drink heavily have an especially high risk of alcohol-related damage.

No matter what your mother may tell you ("I had a cocktail every evening while I was pregnant with you, and you turned out just fine!"), understand that even moderate or light drinking has the potential to harm your baby. *No level of alcohol use during pregnancy has been proven safe.*

Enlisting Support

Don't go it alone—ask your partner to join you as you improve your habits. Tell your partner and anyone else who lives with you how much it would mean to you—and your baby—if they jumped onto the good health bandwagon with you. Think of it as a time to clean up your home environment and start preparing yourself to be great parents.

Using street drugs Street drugs, including cocaine, marijuana, and ecstasy, can cause severe birth defects, miscarriage, or fetal death. If you're using any such drugs, reach out to your provider and ask about programs that can help you quit.

Q: *How often will I have prenatal-care appointments?*

A: *Occasionally at first, and more often as your due date gets closer. Providers usually follow this kind of schedule with healthy women having low-risk pregnancies:*

- **Up to week 28:** *once a month*
- **Weeks 28 through 36:** *every two or three weeks*
- **Weeks 36 through 40:** *every week*
- **Beyond 40 weeks:** *every few days*

Providers usually want to see women with high-risk pregnancies more frequently. Women with other health conditions may also see their specialists at various points during their pregnancy. It's important to keep all scheduled appointments, even if you feel well and your pregnancy is proceeding normally.

Prenatal care isn't something you do just once. You continue to see your prenatal-care provider throughout your pregnancy. Generally, the follow-up visits are shorter than your first one. The goal of these visits is for your provider to check in on you and your baby to make sure everything is going well.

At each appointment, your provider checks your weight and blood pressure, listens to your heart and lungs, tests your urine, and checks in with you about any medical conditions you may have. Your provider also measures your abdomen to make sure your baby is growing properly, listens to your baby's heart rate using a device known as a Doppler fetal monitor, and talks with you about screening tests.

These visits are a great time to ask your provider questions and seek advice on making healthy choices.

Misusing or abusing prescription narcotic painkillers Just because you have a prescription for something doesn't mean it's safe for your baby. Codeine, oxycodone, hydrocodone, and other narcotic painkillers are prescribed legally by doctors to relieve pain. They are safe when used as prescribed by nonpregnant people. But they are *not* safe for pregnant women and should be stopped before pregnancy or as early in pregnancy as possible.

Babies born to women who take these drugs just before conception or in early pregnancy have a higher-than-average rate of several serious birth defects, including congenital heart defects, spina bifida, and congenital glaucoma.

It can be hard to give up painkillers. Fortunately, prenatal providers want to support and help patients quit. If needed, providers can make referrals to programs that offer additional help with quitting.

WHERE TO GIVE BIRTH

Just as you have a choice about what kind of provider to see, you have a choice about where to have your baby—a hospital, a birthing center, or at home. Each has pros and cons that you can consider as you make your decision.

Hospitals Women who want ready access to advanced medical equipment and highly trained specialists typically choose a hospital. If you or your baby has a problem during labor or childbirth in such a facility, emergency help is readily available.

Q: *What is a high-risk pregnancy?*

A: *Most women have low-risk pregnancies without complications. But sometimes a pregnancy is considered "high-risk." This can happen when a woman:*

- *Has high blood pressure, kidney problems, or gestational diabetes (gestational diabetes is diabetes that occurs during gestation, or pregnancy)*
- *Previously gave birth to a preterm or low-birthweight baby or a baby with a birth defect*
- *Has health conditions that need treatment and can complicate pregnancy, such as heart disease, diabetes, or HIV/AIDS*
- *Is pregnant with multiples (twins, triplets, or more)*
- *Has a history of physical or sexual abuse*
- *Is addicted to drugs*
- *Is pregnant with a baby with a birth defect or other health problem*

Many hospitals have neonatal intensive care units (NICUs), which are staffed and equipped to care for babies with serious problems. Women with high-risk pregnancies are often advised to give birth in a hospital with a NICU (usually pronounced *nick*-you) so that the newborn can receive immediate care.

Hospitals tend to use routine fetal monitoring, which some women dislike because it affects their ability to move around during labor. However, an advantage to hospitals is that care is immediately available should an emergency suddenly arise.

Birthing centers In contrast, birthing centers usually have a homier atmosphere. They may be staffed with midwives trained to help women have medication-free births. Birthing centers generally don't have on-staff anesthesiologists available to give epidurals for pain management, although some are able to give other kinds of pain medication during labor.

Q: *Should I deliver my baby in a hospital with a super-high-tech nursery?*

A: *Every hospital with a maternity department must have a nursery—a unit devoted to newborn care. Some provide more extensive care than others. Hospital nurseries are classified by the kind of care they offer:*

- *Level I. Well-newborn nurseries that provide a basic level of medical care to low-risk and healthy newborns*

- *Level II. Special-care nurseries that can care for infants who are moderately ill or born a few weeks early with health problems that are expected to improve rapidly*

- *Level III. Neonatal intensive care units (NICUs) with highly trained providers and advanced equipment to provide complex care, surgery, and life support for infants who are critically ill, very small, or very premature*

If you are having a healthy, low-risk pregnancy, it is not necessary to make special arrangements to give birth in a hospital with a level II or III nursery. However, if you are having pregnancy complications, or your baby has a known or suspected health problem, talk with your provider about whether choosing a hospital with a higher level of newborn care is a good idea.

If you are laboring in a birthing center and things start to get complicated, you may have to be transported to a hospital for a c-section or other medical intervention. Sometimes birthing centers are located within hospitals and you can be transported by stretcher. If not, an ambulance is used for transport. Only women with low-risk pregnancies are good candidates for a birthing center.

If you're not sure which is better for you, ask about seeing the labor and delivery areas in person. Most hospitals and birthing centers offer tours for expectant parents.

Home A very small number of U.S. women opt to give birth at home. Home birth can be comfortable and cozy, because you're in your own environment rather than a medical setting. It's completely understandable that women would rather stay home than go to a hospital or birthing center. Unfortunately, home births carry a two to three times greater risk of newborn death and a much higher risk of complications to the mother if problems occur during delivery. Because of possible risks, the March of Dimes does not recommend giving birth at home.

Chapter Two

How Your Baby Grows

*A month-by-month look at how your baby develops
and how your body changes during pregnancy*

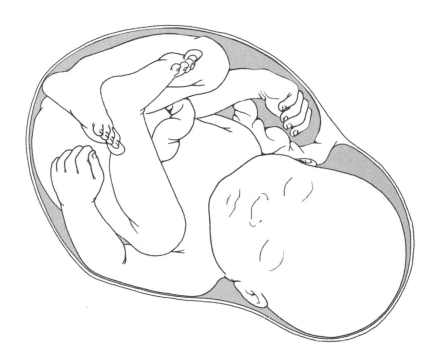

Month 1

Your baby
- Tiny limb buds appear. These grow into your baby's arms and legs.
- Your baby's heart and lungs begin to form. By the 22nd day, your baby's heart starts to beat.
- Your baby's neural tube begins to form. This will become the brain and spinal cord.
- By the end of the first month, your baby is about ¼ inch long.

Your body
- Your body is making lots of hormones that help your baby to grow. Hormones can make you feel moody or cranky.
- Your breasts may get bigger. They may hurt and tingle.
- You may feel sick to your stomach. This is called morning sickness, even though it can happen any time of day. Try eating crackers and smaller meals.
- You may crave some foods or hate foods you usually like.
- You may feel tired. Rest when you can.

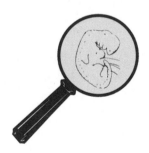

Month 2

Your baby

- Your baby's major body organs, including the brain, the heart, and the lungs, are forming.
- The placenta grows in your uterus and supplies your baby with food and oxygen through the umbilical cord. But you can pass bad things, like alcohol, nicotine, and drugs, through the placenta, too. This is why you want to stay away from alcohol, cigarette smoke, and street drugs when you're pregnant.
- Your baby's ears, ankles, wrists, fingers, and toes are formed. Eyelids form and grow but are sealed shut.
- By the end of the second month, your baby is about 1 inch long and still weighs less than ⅓ ounce.

Your body

- Your breasts may still be sore and are getting bigger. Your nipples and the area around them begin to darken.
- You have to go to the bathroom more often because your uterus is growing and pressing on your bladder.
- You may still have morning sickness.
- You may feel tired and need to rest more often.
- Your body makes more blood.

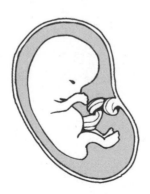

Month 3

Your baby

- Your baby's fingernails and toenails are formed.
- Your baby's mouth has 20 buds that will grow into baby teeth.
- Fine hairs begin to form on your baby's skin.
- With the help of a Doppler fetal monitor (also known as a Doppler), you can hear your baby's heartbeat for the first time. This can be a joyful, exciting moment because it's the first time you really feel that you have a baby inside you.
- By the end of the third month, your baby is 2½ to 3 inches long and weighs about 1 ounce.

Your body

- You may still feel tired and have morning sickness.
- You may have headaches and get lightheaded or dizzy. If these symptoms don't go away, tell your health-care provider. Talk to your provider before you take any medicine for a headache.
- You may have gained 2 to 4 pounds by now. Your clothes may begin to feel tight.

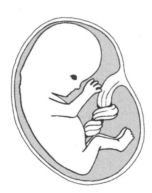

Month 4

Your baby

- Your baby moves, kicks, and swallows.
- Your baby's skin is pink and transparent.
- The placenta is still providing food for your baby. This happens throughout pregnancy. By the end of the fourth month, your baby is 6 to 7 inches long and weighs 4 to 5 ounces.

Your body

- You may get hungrier as your morning sickness goes away. You also might have more energy. But you may start to have heartburn. Try eating four or five smaller meals each day, instead of three larger ones. Avoid spicy foods.
- Near the end of this month, you may feel your baby move for the first time.
- You gain about 1 pound a week. Your belly begins to show. You will probably need to wear maternity clothes and bigger bras now.
- It's okay for you and your partner to have sex if you want. It won't hurt your baby. You may have to try new positions as your belly gets bigger. Do what's comfortable for you.

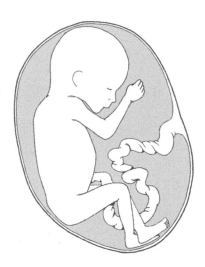

Month 5

Your baby

- Your baby becomes more active and can turn from side to side and sometimes head over heels.
- Your baby goes to sleep and wakes up.
- Your baby grows a lot during this month.
- By the end of the fifth month, your baby is about 10 inches long and weighs ½ to 1 pound.

Your body

- You should feel your baby move inside you this month. If you don't, tell your health-care provider.
- Your heart beats faster.
- You may need eight or more hours of sleep each night. Rest and take breaks during the day if you can. Don't push yourself.

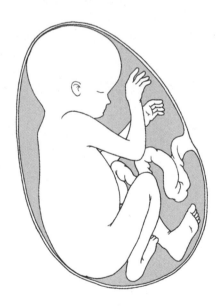

Month 6

Your baby

- Your baby's skin is red and wrinkled. It's covered with fine, soft hair.
- Your baby can kick strongly now.
- Your baby's eyes are almost completely formed. Soon they can start to open and close.
- By the end of the sixth month, your baby is about 12 inches long and weighs 1½ to 2 pounds.

Your body

- The skin on your belly may itch. You may see stretch marks. Use lotion and wear loose clothes.
- Your back may hurt. Don't stand for long periods of time. Don't lift heavy things.
- You may feel pain down the sides of your belly as your uterus gets bigger.
- You may have constipation. Drink more water or fruit juice. Eat more foods with fiber, such as fruits and vegetables.
- You can still have sex, but stop if you feel pain or cramping.

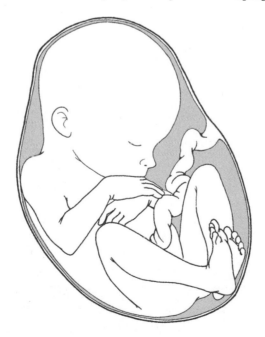

Month 7

Your baby
- Your baby can open and close his or her eyes and suck his or her thumb.
- Your baby kicks and stretches.
- Your baby responds to light and sound.
- By the end of the seventh month, your baby is 15 to 16 inches long and weighs 2½ to 3 pounds.

Your body
- You should feel your baby move. As your baby gets bigger, it may feel like he or she is rolling around. Tell your provider if you notice any change in how often your baby moves.
- Your ankles and feet may swell. Try lying down and putting your feet up. If your hands and face swell suddenly, call your provider.
- You may get additional stretch marks on your belly and breasts as they get bigger.
- You may have occasional contractions. This is okay, but call your provider if you have more than five contractions in one hour.
- As your belly gets bigger, you may find it harder to keep your balance. This makes it easier to fall. Be careful!
- You may have trouble sleeping. Try sleeping on your side or propped up with extra pillows. You may also sweat more than usual.

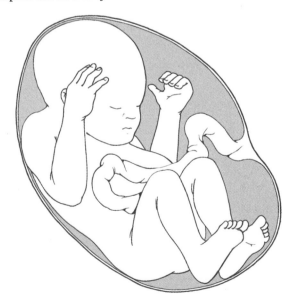

Month 8

Your baby

- Your baby can kick strongly and roll around. You may sometimes see the shape of an elbow or heel against your belly. Tell your provider if you notice any change in how often your baby moves.
- Fingernails have grown to the tips of your baby's fingers.
- Your baby's brain and lungs are still growing.
- By the end of the eighth month, your baby is 18 to 19 inches long and weighs 4 to 5 pounds.

Your body

- You may feel stronger contractions this month.
- Colostrum may leak from your breasts. (This is the fluid that comes out of your breasts before your breast milk comes in.) Wear breast pads in your bra to help with leaking.
- You may have trouble breathing as your baby pushes on your lungs. Slow down, and try to sit and stand up straight.
- Your baby may crowd your stomach. Try eating four or five smaller meals during the day.
- You gain about 1 pound a week this month.

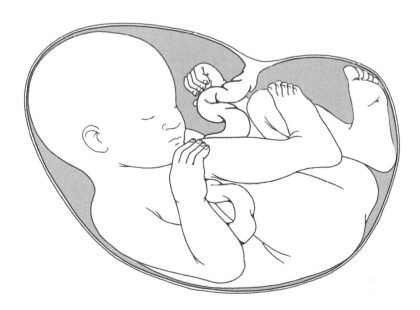

Month 9

Your baby
- Your baby's lungs are ready to work on their own.
- Your baby gains about ½ pound a week.
- Your baby is still moving and kicking.
- Your baby moves to a head-down position and rests lower in your belly.
- By the end of the ninth month, your baby is 19 to 21 inches long and weighs 6 to 9 pounds.

Your body
- Your belly button may stick out.
- Your breathing should be easier once your baby moves down. But you may need to go to the bathroom more often because your baby is pressing on your bladder.
- You should feel your baby kicking and moving right up until you give birth. Tell your provider if you notice any change in how often your baby moves.
- You may be uncomfortable because of the pressure and weight of your baby. Rest often.
- Your feet and ankles may swell. Put your feet up. Try to stay in a cool place.
- Your cervix opens up (dilates) and thins out (effaces) as it prepares for birth.
- You may not gain any weight this month. You may even lose 1 or 2 pounds.

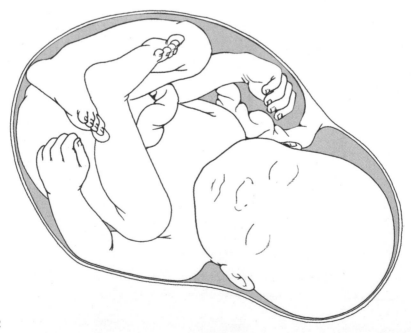

Chapter Three

What to Eat

Pregnancy is a great opportunity to change the way you think about food. Like many women, you may have followed crazy diets or made poor eating choices at various times in your life. Who hasn't gone overboard on junk food and skipped meals to make up for it? Who hasn't relied too heavily on greasy fast food instead of taking the time to make healthy meals?

Many women have lived this way for so long that they're not even sure *how* to eat healthfully. If that's you, don't worry. You can learn and change. Your goal over the next few months is to choose nutritious foods, avoid anything that could harm your baby, and eat the right amount of food. You don't have to make all these changes at once. You can start small, by changing one or two things at a time.

Improving your diet during pregnancy is an excellent dress rehearsal for feeding your baby. Begin making smart changes in your daily menu now, and by the time your baby starts eating solid foods you'll be a seasoned expert with loads of experience in choosing and preparing nutritious foods. You'll be all set to pass your own healthy eating habits on to your child!

BECOMING A HEALTHY ROLE MODEL

Eating for optimal health in pregnancy isn't just about avoiding certain foods, although there are a few foods to stay away from for safety reasons. To start with, healthy eating means making the best possible food choices most of the time. It also means opening up to new tastes and flavors, trying new foods, eating more unprocessed foods, and appreciating how delicious health-promoting foods can be. As you eat to fuel your pregnancy, you can also eat for pleasure and enjoyment.

Think of improving your diet as a process, something you can work on each day that can have wonderful rewards for you and your baby now and for the rest of your life.

One easy change to make is simply to pay more attention to your food. If you're used to wolfing down food so fast that you barely taste it, simply slowing down and being mindful of what you're eating can increase your enjoyment of it.

You'll be amazed at how much difference it makes to really focus on the taste and texture of food—the juicy sweet-tartness of an apple, the satisfying crunch of a crispy-fresh salad, the rich burst of earthy-sweet richness in a fabulous piece of dark chocolate. When you stop and pay attention to what you eat, you can enjoy it more and improve your relationship with food in a healthy, satisfying way.

How much do you need to change your diet during pregnancy? If you're already eating healthfully, you may need to make only a few minor tweaks. If you haven't eaten a piece of fruit since third grade, you probably need more of an overhaul. Either way, focus on small changes you can make today. Gradual change will be more successful in the long term than an all-at-once change.

ESSENTIAL NUTRITION

Food contains a range of different vitamins, minerals, and other nutrients that your body needs to live and thrive. For example, vitamin C helps wounds heal. Vitamin D and calcium help bones stay strong. Vitamin E helps protect cells from damage. Iron helps blood deliver oxygen to all of your body's cells.

During pregnancy, you need a little more of certain nutrients because of all the extra work your body is doing. You can make sure you're getting enough of each important nutrient by taking your prenatal multivitamin and including nutritious foods in your menu every day.

The following nutrients are especially important during pregnancy:

Folate/folic acid This B vitamin is crucial before and during pregnancy to reduce the risk of neural tube defects. (It is called folate in foods, and folic acid in supplements.) Although folate is found in foods such as dark leafy greens and dried beans, supplements are recommended as extra insurance to make sure you get the folic acid you need. Be sure you're taking a supplement with 600 to 800 micrograms of folic acid—or more if your provider recommends it.

Calcium Your body uses calcium to build and maintain bones and teeth in your body and your baby's. Calcium also helps keep blood vessels and nerves healthy. Getting plenty of calcium during pregnancy is critical, because if you don't, your body takes calcium from your bones to meet your baby's calcium needs—and that can raise your chances of bone thinning and osteoporosis later in life.

Dairy foods such as milk, yogurt, and cheese are excellent sources of calcium. However, full-fat versions of these foods are high in saturated fat, which is not good for your heart. Whenever possible, choose low-fat or nonfat versions. Nondairy sources of calcium include broccoli, dark leafy greens such as spinach, canned salmon, and sardines with bones.

If you have trouble getting the calcium you need from your diet, talk with your provider about taking additional calcium supplements. (Prenatal vitamins usually contain only about one-quarter of your daily calcium requirement, so they can't make up for the calcium shortfall in a dairy-free diet.)

Vitamin D This vitamin is important because it helps your body use calcium. It is not found naturally in many foods, so it is often added to calcium-rich foods such as milk. Your body can also manufacture its own vitamin D in the presence of sunlight.

Researchers say that as many as half of Americans don't get enough vitamin D. Among women of childbearing age, those most likely to be low on vitamin D are obese women, women who spend little time outdoors (especially darker-skinned women, because sunlight penetrates darker skin more slowly), and women with digestive disorders such as Crohn's disease or celiac disease that prevent them from absorbing nutrients well.

Iron Iron helps your blood carry oxygen to all your cells. During pregnancy, when your blood volume increases by 50 percent, you need iron to build new blood for yourself and your baby. Also, iron from your body is stored in your baby's body for use during your baby's first few months of life.

Too little iron can cause anemia, which raises the risk of preterm birth and having a low-birthweight baby. Your provider can test your blood to see if it contains enough iron. If your iron is low, you may be advised to take an iron supplement in addition to your prenatal multivitamin.

THE BUILDING BLOCKS OF FOOD

Food contains protein, carbohydrates, and fats.

Protein Your body uses the protein in food to build and maintain your growing baby's tissues and organs, as well as your placenta and the additional blood your body manufactures while you're pregnant. After you've given birth, your body uses protein to make milk for breastfeeding.

Your body needs ample protein during pregnancy, but there's no need to go overboard by eating a high-protein diet.

Recommended intake. The average pregnant woman needs about 71 grams of protein per day—about 50 percent more than nonpregnant women.

Good sources. Meat, fish, eggs, milk, cheese, dried beans, lentils, split peas, nuts, and seeds.

Carbohydrates Carbohydrates provide your body with fuel. There are two kinds of carbohydrates: complex carbohydrates (starches) and simple carbohydrates (sugars). Your body breaks carbohydrates down into glucose (a form of sugar), which your blood carries throughout your body to give energy to all of your cells. Glucose that is not immediately used is eventually converted to animal starch (glycogen) and stored for future use.

In general, it's best to choose foods with complex carbohydrates (such as whole-grain bread) because they tend to contain more nutrients than highly processed foods with lots of simple carbohydrates (such as white bread). Complex carbohydrates help keep blood sugar levels even because they break down slowly; simple carbohydrates can cause blood sugar to spike. In addition, complex carbohydrates are often high in fiber, which helps move food through the digestive system. Fiber can be a woman's best friend if she has constipation, a common discomfort during pregnancy.

Recommended intake. Pregnant women need about 175 grams of carbohydrates, including at least 28 grams of fiber per day.

Good sources. Whole-grain bread and cereal, fruits, vegetables, rice, and tortillas.

Fats Your body uses fats for storing energy, building healthy cells, keeping your body warm, and making hormones. Fats also help your body absorb and store vitamins A, D, E, and K, which are known as fat-soluble vitamins. There are several kinds of fats:

- **Unsaturated.** These fats are often called "good" fats because they contribute to heart health. There are two kinds of unsaturated fats: polyunsaturated and monounsaturated. Sources of polyunsaturated fat include certain cooking oils (such as safflower, sunflower, and corn) and nuts. Sources of monounsaturated fats include olive oil, canola oil, nuts, salmon, and avocados.

- **Saturated.** Commonly known as "bad" fats, saturated fats can raise heart disease risk. Foods high in saturated fats include fatty meats, full-fat cheese, whole milk, butter, and tropical oils (palm, coconut, and palm kernel).

- **Trans.** Also known as trans-fatty acids, trans fats are another category of "bad" fat. They are created when unsaturated fats are processed and chemically changed from liquid to solid form. Sources of trans fats, which raise heart disease risk, include shortening, many margarines, some commercially prepared fried foods, and packaged baked goods, crackers, and snack foods.

Recommended intake. Pregnant women should get 20 to 35 percent of their calories from fat. For a woman with a daily goal of 2,200 calories, that's 48 to 85 grams of fat per day.

Good sources. Most of the fats you eat should be unsaturated, from sources such as nuts, avocados, and olive oil.

IMPORTANT VITAMINS AND MINERALS

Although your prenatal vitamin delivers many of the vitamins and minerals you and your baby need, it's still necessary to eat food sources of these nutrients. This chart shows how various nutrients help you and your baby, and lists good food sources of the nutrients for pregnant women age 19 and older.

Nutrient	Some of the body parts that need it	Good food sources
Vitamin A	Skin, eyes, bones	Eggs, fish, many yellow, red, and orange fruits and vegetables (sweet potatoes, carrots, tomatoes, apricots), dark leafy greens such as spinach and kale

Nutrient	Some of the body parts that need it	Good food sources
Thiamin (B$_1$)	Brain, nerves, heart	Whole grains, dried beans, lean meats, nuts
Riboflavin (B$_2$)	Blood, skin, eyes	Dairy products, red meat, chicken, fish, dark leafy greens, nuts, eggs
Niacin (B$_3$)	Skin, nerves, digestive system	Nuts, grains, red meat, fish, chicken
Vitamin B$_6$ (pyridoxine)	Brain, immune system; also helps body use protein and glucose	Whole grains, fortified breakfast cereals, bananas, red meat, beans, nuts, chicken, fish
Vitamin B$_{12}$	Blood, nerves	Beef, pork, poultry, eggs, dairy
Folate	Cells; helps build DNA and RNA	Fortified breakfast cereals, enriched breads and grain products, beans, dark leafy greens, orange juice
Vitamin C	Gums, teeth; helps body absorb iron, heal wounds	Citrus fruits, strawberries, bell peppers, broccoli
Vitamin D	Bones, teeth; helps calcium do its job	Milk, salmon, orange juice, fortified breakfast cereals
Vitamin E	Immune system, blood vessels; protects cells from damage	Nuts, vegetable oils, wheat germ, dark leafy greens, seeds, whole grains
Vitamin K	Bones; also helps with blood clotting	Cauliflower, broccoli, dark leafy greens, cabbage, milk, soybeans, eggs
Calcium	Bones and teeth, muscles and nerves; helps blood clot normally	Low-fat and nonfat dairy products (milk, yogurt, cheese), calcium-fortified soy milk, calcium-fortified orange juice, canned salmon and sardines with bones, dark leafy greens (though calcium in vegetables is not absorbed as readily as calcium in dairy foods)
Magnesium	Muscles, nerves, heart, immune system, bones	Halibut, almonds, cashews, soybeans, spinach, potatoes, peanuts, black-eyed peas, yogurt, legumes, fortified breakfast cereals
Iron	Blood, muscles; helps blood deliver oxygen throughout the body	Lean red meat, dried beans and peas, fortified breakfast cereals, dark leafy greens, peanuts
Zinc	Cells; helps with cell growth, wound repair, immune system	Oysters, crabmeat, eggs, poultry, wheat germ, dried beans, whole grains, nuts

WHAT'S ON YOUR PLATE?

It's good to know about the nutrients your body needs during pregnancy. But since you eat *food*, not *nutrients*, let's take a look at some of the best foods for you to eat while you're pregnant.

Great Grains: Bread, Cereal, Pasta, and Rice

Why you need them Grains contain a variety of nutrients, including several B vitamins, fiber, iron, and magnesium. The best grains for human health are whole grains, which help prevent constipation, a common problem during pregnancy, and help keep blood sugar levels stable. Refined grains (white bread, white pasta, and white rice) are less nutritious because the refining process removes certain nutrients—although some are added back during manufacturing.

Best choices Brown rice, oatmeal, unbuttered popcorn, barley, and quinoa, as well as breakfast cereals, bread, crackers, pasta, rice, bagels, tortillas, cornbread, and noodles made with whole grains or whole-grain flour.

Eating to Soothe

Certain foods can help ease these pregnancy discomforts:

Morning sickness. *Try nibbling on crackers, bread, or cereal before getting out of bed in the morning. In addition, try eating five or six smaller meals a day instead of three bigger ones, and cut back on foods that are greasy, spicy, or highly aromatic.*

Constipation. *Drinking plenty of water and eating high-fiber foods such as whole grains, legumes, fruits, and vegetables can help get things moving within you.*

Diarrhea. *Try the so-called BRAT diet, which stands for bananas, rice, applesauce, and toast.*

Heartburn. *You may find relief by avoiding caffeine, eating smaller meals, avoiding foods that are greasy and spicy, and remaining upright (not lying down) for at least an hour or so after eating. Some women find that plain yogurt cools the burn.*

How much to have Aim for 6 ounces per day in the first trimester, 7 ounces in the second trimester, and 8 ounces in the third trimester. One ounce of grains is equal to:

- 1 slice bread

- 1 cup ready-to-eat dry cereal

- ½ cup cooked rice, pasta, or cereal

- 1 small pancake (4½ inches in diameter)

- 1 small tortilla (6 inches in diameter)

A Rainbow of Vegetables

Why you need them Vegetables provide lots of vitamins, minerals, and fiber. Nutrients are often found in vegetable pigments, with different colors offering different benefits. For example, yellow and orange vegetables help promote eye health.

IN DEPTH
Nutrition Requirements for Pregnant Teens
See page 245

Best choices Dark-green vegetables (spinach, watercress, kale, bok choy, broccoli, romaine lettuce), red and orange vegetables (bell peppers, tomatoes, squash, carrots, sweet potatoes), starchy vegetables (corn, cassava, potatoes, plantains, taro, green peas), and other vegetables (asparagus, zucchini, Brussels sprouts, lettuce, and cucumbers).

Beans and lentils, which are generally considered vegetables even though they belong to the legume family, also contain lots of protein.

How much to have Aim for 2½ cups per day in the first trimester and 3 cups per day in the second and third trimesters. One cup of vegetables is equal to:

- 1 cup raw or cooked vegetables

- 1 cup vegetable juice (which can be very salty, so choose low-sodium varieties)

- 2 cups raw dark leafy greens

- 1 medium baked potato

- 1 cup cooked legumes

Give Beans a Chance

We get it. Beans don't make it onto many people's favorite-foods list. But if you're not eating beans on a regular basis, you're missing out on a fabulous food. Beans and other legumes are packed with nutrients that are crucial for pregnant women and their babies, such as protein, B vitamins (including folate), magnesium, fiber, zinc, and iron.

Members of the legume family include all kinds of beans, black-eyed peas, chickpeas (also called garbanzo beans), soy nuts, and lentils.

These super-nutritious foods are inexpensive and simple to prepare. Canned beans are especially easy to stir into favorite recipes such as soups, salads, chili, stew, and rice and pasta dishes. Try mashing some drained canned white beans with garlic, olive oil, and lemon juice, and you have a quick, tasty dip for fresh vegetables. Or toss together drained canned beans, Italian dressing, and chopped red onions for a delicious bean salad.

Legumes provide many of the nutrients found in meat, so they're an excellent meat substitute for vegetarians and people who choose to cut back on their meat intake.

Legumes are equally nutritious whether you buy them uncooked (dried), canned, or frozen. Some canned varieties contain salt, but rinsing them with water washes most of it away.

Powerful Protein: Meat, Fish, Eggs, and Beans

Why you need it Protein contributes to the healthy growth and functioning of cells, tissues, and organs in your body and your baby's body. Pregnant women need about 50 percent more protein than nonpregnant women: protein is necessary for the healthy growth and functioning of a baby's cells, tissues, brain, muscles, blood, and organs, as well as for the placenta, amniotic fluid, and extra maternal blood.

Best choices Lean meats (beef, chicken, turkey, lamb, and pork), seafood, eggs, soy-based foods, nuts, and seeds. And don't forget protein-packed beans.

How much to have Aim for 5 ounces per day in the first trimester, 6 ounces per day in the second trimester, and 6½ ounces per day in the third trimester. One ounce of protein is equal to:

- 1 tablespoon peanut butter
- ¼ cup cooked beans
- 1 ounce lean meat, poultry, or fish
- 1 egg
- ½ ounce nuts (12 almonds, 24 pistachios)

A Sweet Selection of Fruits

Why you need them Fruits offer a wide range of nutrients. As with vegetables, fruits of different colors provide a mix of vitamins and minerals.

Best choices Apples, bananas, berries, cherries, citrus fruits, dried fruits, grapes, kiwis, melons, peaches, pears, papayas, pineapples, mangos, and fruit juices (but only those that are 100 percent pure juice).

How much to have Aim for 1½ to 2 cups per day in the first trimester and 2 cups per day in the second and third trimesters. Half a cup of fruit is equal to:

- ½ cup 100 percent fruit juice (limit your juice intake because it's high in natural sugar, which can send blood sugar levels soaring)
- ½ cup fresh, frozen, or canned fruit

Power Bars and Energy Drinks: A Good Source of Protein?

Grocery shelves are well stocked with power bars and energy drinks. These processed products usually contain a fair amount of protein, but they may also be packed with sugar, unhealthy fats, calories, and excessive amounts of vitamins and minerals. Food in its natural state is a better source of protein. Having a protein bar once in a while is fine, but try to leave it at that. Peanut butter on whole-grain bread is almost as convenient as a power bar, and that combination provides protein, fiber, and other nutrients in a less-processed form.

- ½ small orange, apple, or banana
- ¼ cup dried fruit
- 16 grapes

Bone-Building Dairy Foods: Milk, Cheese, and Yogurt

Why you need them Dairy foods contain protein and calcium; some also have
vitamin D. They are very important for bone health.

Best choices Milk, cheese, yogurt, ice cream, and puddings and soups made
with milk or calcium-fortified soy milk. When possible, choose heart-healthy
reduced fat or nonfat dairy foods.

If dairy bothers you Milk contains lactose, a sugar that in some people can
cause diarrhea, cramping, and gas. If you have trouble tolerating lactose, try
drinking milk in small amounts with food or replacing milk with yogurt and
cheese, which may cause fewer problems. If those solutions don't work, drink
lactose-free milk.

How much to have Aim for 3 cups per day throughout pregnancy. One cup
of dairy is equal to:

- 1 cup milk
- 1 cup calcium-fortified soy milk
- 1 cup lactose-free milk

- 1 cup yogurt
- 2 small slices of cheese or ⅓ cup shredded cheese

Don't Forget Fats: Oils, Fatty Fish, and Nuts

Why you need them Fats help your body store energy, build healthy cells, keep warm, and make hormones. Fats also help your body absorb and store certain vitamins.

Best choices Heart-healthy unsaturated and monounsaturated fats such as certain cooking oils (olive, canola, sunflower, safflower, corn), fatty fish, nuts,

Food for Thought: Omega-3 Fatty Acids

Omega-3 fatty acids are a family of fats that are especially important for pregnant women.

There are three major omega-3 fatty acids: ALA, EPA, and DHA. (Those letters stand for nutritional compounds, but unless you're a dietitian, you don't need to know more than just the letters.)

Omega-3 fatty acids are good for you and your baby. They help with your baby's brain and eye health. DHA is especially important during the third trimester, when your baby's brain is growing rapidly.

Most people get plenty of ALA, which is found in vegetable oils, walnuts, and some green vegetables, such as spinach. DHA and EPA are a little harder to get, because they're found primarily in fish, including salmon, herring, sardines, and white tuna. (Unfortunately, some of the fish we eat today is contaminated with mercury. For information about mercury in fish, see the conclusion of this chapter.)

Pregnant women should get at least 200 milligrams of DHA each day, but most fall short, getting only 60 to 80 milligrams daily. You can get the DHA you need by eating two servings (a total of 12 ounces) of fish each week. (There is no specific recommendation for ALA or EPA.) If you don't eat fish, talk with your provider about taking DHA supplements that are safe for pregnant women. Avoid supplements that are made from fish liver, because they may contain unacceptably high levels of vitamin A.

and avocados. Avoid less-healthy fats such as saturated fat (found in animal products such as meat and full-fat cheese, ice cream, milk, and other dairy) and trans fat (found in shortening and many commercially prepared cookies, cakes, crackers, and fried foods), which are not good for your heart.

How to Eat Well on a Budget

Fresh fruits and vegetables are packed with vitamins and other good things that can help keep you and your baby healthy. But they can be expensive. Here are some tips to help you shop for nutritious foods without spending a lot of money:

- *Make a budget and a menu for the week. Check store flyers to see what's on sale, and create your menu around those items. See what you already have at home, and then make a list of what you need to buy. Stick to the list when you're at the store.*

- *Shop around, checking out larger grocery stores, the farmers' market, and/ or farm stands. They may have better prices for fresh foods than smaller grocery stores in your neighborhood.*

- *Find out if your store has a discount card. It can help you save money on food and other products. Most discount cards are free, so get one for every store in your area.*

- *Compare prices between store brands and name brands. Often the store brands cost less.*

- *Buy whole fruits and vegetables. The ones that come already washed and cut cost more.*

- *Buy canned or frozen fruits and vegetables, which with today's processing techniques retain most of their nutrients. Avoid added sugar in fruit by choosing unsweetened frozen fruit or canned fruit that's packed in its own juice.*

- *Make more than you need, and freeze the extra for future meals. Also, freeze unused vegetables and herbs such as onions, peppers, garlic, and parsley.*

- *Have a meatless meal now and then, since meat is the most expensive thing on your grocery list. For example, try rice and beans or vegetable lasagna.*

- *Keep staple foods—items that you can use for almost any meal—on hand. Examples are beans, rice, pasta, frozen vegetables, pasta sauce, and peanut butter.*

How much to have There's no across-the-board recommendation for fat. Experts say we should all get 20 to 35 percent of our calories from fat. For a woman with a daily goal of 2,200 calories, that's 48 to 85 grams of fat per day—the equivalent of about 3½ to 6 tablespoons of oil. Most should be unsaturated.

For Caffeine Addicts

Women who love their morning coffee hate the idea of giving it up when they get pregnant. Must you go nine months without a drop of caffeine?

No. Although large amounts of caffeine may contribute to risk of miscarriage and preterm birth, smaller amounts seem to be safe. Recommendations suggest that you limit yourself to 200 milligrams of caffeine per day. That's the amount in about one 12-ounce cup of coffee. But remember to include all other sources of caffeine too, including tea, soda, and chocolate.

Keep in mind that caffeine can worsen heartburn and reduce iron absorption when it's consumed with foods that contain iron, such as lean beef and leafy green vegetables. If you've got heartburn or anemia, you may want to further limit caffeine intake and opt for caffeine-free foods and decaffeinated drinks instead.

The following list shows the amount of caffeine in several foods and drinks. Keep in mind, however, that the amount of caffeine in brewed drinks such as coffee and tea can vary widely depending on how a specific portion is made. Some coffee shops brew exceptionally strong beverages. The stronger the drink, the higher its caffeine content.

Caffeine is also found in some headache, pain, and cold medications. Check the label before taking these medications so you know what you're taking.

Food	Caffeine content in milligrams
Milk chocolate (1 ounce)	1–15
Cola (12 ounces)	25–65
Hot cocoa and chocolate milk	0–20
Coffee (8 ounces brewed)	100–150
Tea (brewed with one tea bag)	80

HUNGRY FOR ANSWERS

Pregnant women think a lot about what they should (and shouldn't) eat and drink. Here are answers to some of their most common questions:

Q: *What should I do about food cravings—give in to them, or just wait for them to go away?*

A: Food cravings are completely normal during pregnancy—most women have them at some point. It's fine to eat a food you crave, provided you do so in moderation and it doesn't interfere with your healthy diet.

If you crave junk food, try eating a small amount of the food and see if that satisfies you. In other words, if you're dying for fast-food french fries, don't buy the supersize. Instead, get a small order and eat them slowly or share them with a friend. Eating a small serving mindfully often satisfies your craving better than a large amount gobbled up without much thought.

Some pregnant women have a strong urge to eat things that are not food, such as clay, cornstarch, laundry starch, or soil—a condition called pica. Pica can cause serious problems for your health. Pregnant women should never eat nonfood items, so if you feel the urge to, talk with your provider about it.

Q: *Should I cut down on salt?*

A: Your pregnant body does need some sodium, a mineral found in salt. Sodium helps your body keep a healthy fluid balance. It also helps keep muscles, nerves, and blood healthy. If your kidneys are working well, they get rid of excess salt. Even so, most Americans eat much more salt than they need. It's best to go easy with the salt shaker and with foods that are high in salt, including snack foods such as chips and pretzels, canned soups, and frozen dinners. There can also be surprisingly high amounts of salt in salad dressings, vegetable juices, spaghetti sauces, lunch meats, condiments, and spice mixes.

Q: *I don't want my baby to have food allergies. Can I lower the risk by staying away from allergy-causing foods?*

A: Unless you have food allergies yourself, there's no reason to avoid the eight foods that account for 90 percent of food allergies: milk, eggs, peanuts, tree nuts, fish, shellfish, soy, and wheat. There's no proof that skipping these foods lowers your baby's allergy risk later in life—in fact, some studies suggest that eating them during pregnancy may actually help prevent food allergies in your baby.

These foods are nutritious—for example, the fats in fish and shellfish contribute to your baby's brain development, and the folate in peanuts lowers the risk of neural tube defects—so avoiding them appears to do more harm than good.

Q: *Are herbal teas safe?*

A: Certain herbs are more powerful than you would expect—for example, the herb passionflower contains chemicals that can cause the uterus to contract. Little research has been done on the safety or medical effects of many herbs. Furthermore, herbal products are not well regulated. For these reasons, it's best to avoid herbal teas during pregnancy—even those on grocery-store shelves.

Q: *Are artificial sweeteners safe?*

A: Sugar substitutes such as acesulfame potassium, aspartame, saccharin, neotame, and sucralose are thought to be safe to eat in moderate amounts during pregnancy.

Saccharin may cause bladder cancer in rats when ingested in high doses, but the U.S. Food and Drug Administration says humans are not in danger. Saccharin does cross the placenta and can accumulate in your baby's body, so its consumption during pregnancy is controversial. The most cautious choice is to avoid it.

Note: Women with a metabolic disorder known as phenylketonuria (PKU) should not have aspartame (sold as NutraSweet or Equal) because it contains an ingredient (phenylalanine) that their bodies cannot process.

Q: *May I have an occasional glass of wine or beer while I'm pregnant? I can't imagine that one drink would do any harm.*

A: There is *no* amount of alcohol that has been proven to be safe during pregnancy—even small amounts could harm your baby's developing nervous system. Pour a glass of sparkling water, fruit juice mixed with club soda, or nonalcoholic beer or wine, or make a delicious alcohol-free mocktail instead. Drinking even small amounts of alcohol is not a risk worth taking.

Q: *Is it better to drink bottled water instead of tap water?*

A: Unless your tap water contains lead or other unsafe contaminants, you don't need to switch to bottled water. Some women are concerned about the safety of chemicals used to make certain kinds of plastic containers that bottled water is sold in; they worry that those chemicals may contaminate the contents. Also, most tap water is supplemented with fluoride, a mineral that contributes to the health of your baby's teeth and lowers your risk of tooth decay and gum disease. Relying only on bottled water may prevent you from getting the fluoride you and your baby need. If you drink bottled water or if your tap water does not contain fluoride, talk with your provider about using fluoride supplements. For more on drinking water safety and plastics safety, see chapter 8.

Q: *How much water should I drink?*

A: Each day, most people need about 64 ounces (about eight glasses) of water, which can come from food and drinks. You may need more when it's hot out or if you exercise or are constipated. Generally, if you drink when you're thirsty, you get all the water you need. Whenever possible, opt for water over sweet drinks such as soda, sweetened ice tea, and fruit punches. Or, flavor water with a squeeze of fresh lemon, lime, or orange.

If vomiting caused by morning sickness prevents you from getting enough water, you may be at risk of dehydration, which can be harmful to you and your baby. Call your provider if you're having trouble staying hydrated.

Q: *Do I really have to heat up lunch meat, stay away from homemade cheese, give up sushi, and stop eating raw cookie dough batter?*

A: Unfortunately, you do. These and other steps help protect you from foodborne infections that can be surprisingly dangerous to you and your baby. Read on to find out more.

AVOIDING FOOD-BORNE INFECTIONS AND TOXINS

Ick. Who wants to read about food-borne infections? Nobody. But you need to know about them. Food-borne infections can make you sick and hurt your baby.

Various kinds of germs can cause food-borne infections. They can bring on unpleasant gastrointestinal symptoms such as diarrhea, vomiting, and abdominal cramps, as well as muscle aches and fever. These germs spread when food is handled improperly at home, during food processing, and in restaurants. Some infections happen when food isn't cooked or stored properly; others occur when food handlers don't keep their hands, utensils, and preparation surfaces clean enough.

There are lots of simple steps you can take to protect yourself and your baby from food-borne infections. The first one is learning about how to prevent foods from becoming unsafe and how to protect yourself from contaminated food.

Listeriosis

No, it's not a mouthwash. It's an infection that can cause big problems if you're not careful. But it's easy to avoid if you know how.

Listeriosis is caused by a bacterium in the genus *Listeria*, which may be found in unpasteurized milk, cheese, and fruit juice. (Pasteurization is a heating process used to kill bacteria—read food labels to check for pasteurization.) It may also be found in some refrigerated ready-to-eat foods, unwashed fruits and vegetables, and undercooked meat, poultry, and seafood, as well as garden soil.

Most healthy adults don't get sick if they eat foods tainted with *Listeria*. But pregnant women are more susceptible to *Listeria* infection and are 20 times more likely than other adults to develop listeriosis.

Listeriosis during pregnancy can cause preterm labor, low birthweight, miscarriage, stillbirth, and serious health problems in a baby. It can be treated with antibiotics, but treatment doesn't eliminate all risks. It's safest to avoid infection.

Protect yourself from *Listeria*

- Cook all meat, seafood, poultry, and eggs thoroughly. Don't eat raw or undercooked fish or shellfish, including sushi and sashimi.

- Use separate knives and cutting boards for raw meat and cooked meat.

- Cook eggs until both the yolk and white are firm. Do not eat foods that contain eggs that are not fully cooked, such as eggnog, some kinds of mousse, meringue made with raw egg whites, raw cookie dough, and hollandaise sauce. (Pasteurized raw egg products are available in some grocery stores—try using them instead.)

- Order meats in restaurants to be cooked medium well or well done. If food seems inadequately cooked, send it back.

- If you marinate raw meat, throw the marinade away. Do not brush it on cooking meat.

- Don't drink unpasteurized milk, apple cider, or other drinks.

- If you like soft cheeses such as queso fresco, queso blanco, panela, feta, brie, camembert, and blue cheese, choose types that are pasteurized.

- In the grocery store, cover your hand with a plastic bag while handling meat packages that may be contaminated with the juices of raw meats. Then use the bag to enclose the meat package so juices won't leak onto your other groceries.

- Don't eat refrigerated smoked meats and fish (such as lox or kippers), pâté, or meat spread. (Canned varieties are fine because they are heated during the canning process.)

- High temperatures kill *Listeria*, so heat hotdogs and deli meats such as ham, turkey, salami, and bologna until they steam.

- To prevent the growth of bacteria on foods, set your refrigerator to 40°F (or below) and your freezer to 0°F (or below). Use a thermometer to verify refrigerator and freezer temperatures.

- Do not leave meats, cheeses, and other foods that can go bad at room temperature for more than two hours (or one hour if it's over 90°F in the room). Refrigerate or freeze leftovers promptly.

Salmonellosis

Bacteria in the genus *Salmonella* can cause an infection called salmonellosis. Foods contaminated with *Salmonella* tend to be animal foods (beef, milk, poultry, eggs, pork), although other foods such as fruits, vegetables, and even nuts can carry these bacteria as well. Contamination occurs when people who handle foods don't wash their hands well with soap after using the bathroom, or when foods come in contact with sewage.

Salmonella may also be found in the feces of pets, especially turtles, lizards, snakes, frogs, and birds.

There's typically no treatment for *Salmonella* infection, but supportive care such as fluids, rest, and medication for vomiting, fever, and diarrhea may be given. Be sure to call your provider if you think you have been infected.

Protect yourself from *Salmonella*

- Don't eat raw vegetable sprouts (alfalfa, clover, radish, and mung bean).

- Wash your hands thoroughly after using the bathroom, changing a baby's diaper, or having any contact with animals, birds, and reptiles, and insist that members of your household do also.

- Wash fruits and vegetables well before eating.

- Pay attention to news reports about salmonellosis outbreaks, and avoid foods that may be contaminated.

E. coli Infection

Escherichia coli—commonly known as *E. coli*—is a type of bacterium that can cause diarrhea, vomiting, abdominal pain, and sometimes fever. Outbreaks of *E. coli* infection have occurred as a result of contamination of ground beef, vegetable sprouts, unpasteurized fruit juices, dry-cured salami, lettuce, game meat, cheese curds, and unpasteurized milk. *E. coli* can also be found in animal feces. In pregnant women, *E. coli* infection may increase risk of miscarriage or preterm delivery.

Protect yourself from *E. coli*

- To protect yourself from *E. coli* infection, follow the safe food-handling practices listed in the listeriosis section, pay attention to news reports about outbreaks of contaminated foods, and avoid anything that might be unsafe.

Wash, Wash, Wash

Soap and water are two of your best tools for protecting yourself from food-borne infections. Be sure to wash your hands thoroughly before handling food and after touching raw meat, fish, eggs, or poultry. Wash preparation surfaces, knives, and other utensils in hot, soapy water after contact with raw meat. Wash fruits and vegetables well before eating them. Finally, wash your hands thoroughly after using the bathroom, changing a baby's diaper, touching pets, gardening, or doing yard work. A little bit of caution (along with some soap and water) can go a long way toward keeping you and your baby safe.

Use Your Thermometer

Like most cooks, you probably decide if meat is cooked enough simply by cutting a piece open and looking at it. Your meat thermometer most likely comes out of the drawer only at Thanksgiving.

You may want to start thinking of your meat thermometer as a tool for a healthy pregnancy. Cooking meat and poultry thoroughly kills most germs that can cause illness. But eyeballing meat isn't a great way to tell if it's cooked enough. Sometimes meat can look fully cooked even if it isn't.

Use a meat thermometer to make sure your meats are cooked to these temperatures:

- *Pork roasts and chops, beef, veal, lamb roasts, and steaks: at least 145°F*
- *Ground beef, veal, lamb, and pork: at least 160°F*
- *Ground poultry: at least 165°F*
- *Chicken breasts: at least 170°F*
- *Whole poultry: at least 180°F*

Toxoplasmosis

Toxoplasmosis is your ticket to a nine-month vacation from cleaning your cat's litter box. It's caused by *Toxoplasma gondii,* a parasite found in raw and undercooked meat and poultry, unwashed fruits and vegetables, and cat feces in litter boxes and outdoor soil.

If you develop toxoplasmosis while you're pregnant, your baby is at risk of intellectual disabilities, hearing loss, and blindness. Symptoms of toxoplasmosis can include fever, headache, swollen glands, muscle aches, and neck stiffness.

Protect yourself from toxoplasmosis

- When handling raw meat, follow the safe food-handling guidelines listed in the listeriosis section, and keep meat and meat juices away from utensils and from food that will not be cooked.

- Wear gloves while gardening.

- If you have a cat, ask someone else to clean the litter box. If you must do it, wear gloves and wash your hands well afterward. It's best to have the litter box changed every day.

- Keep children's sandboxes covered—outdoor cats like to use them as litter boxes.

- Avoid feeding your cat raw meat.

- Avoid touching stray cats and kittens.

- Avoid adopting a new cat or kitten during pregnancy.

PROS AND CONS OF SEAFOOD

Seafood has pluses and minuses for pregnant women.

On the one hand, it's full of important nutrients, including fats that help babies develop a healthy brain. Fish and shellfish are good sources of protein and omega-3 fatty acids such as brain-building DHA.

On the other hand, some kinds of fish and shellfish contain high levels of mercury, which can damage your baby's nervous system and cause brain damage, learning disabilities, and hearing loss.

So what should you do?

The U.S. Food and Drug Administration and the Environmental Protection Agency have come up with fish-eating guidelines that try to balance the risks and benefits of eating seafood. Basically, these guidelines suggest eating small amounts of some kinds of fish and completely avoiding others.

Here are the guidelines:

- Do not eat fish that may contain high levels of mercury: shark, swordfish, king mackerel, and tilefish.

- Limit your weekly fish intake to no more than 12 ounces total (two average meals) of fish and shellfish that may contain low levels of mercury, including shrimp, salmon, pollock, catfish, and light canned tuna. White albacore tuna may have more mercury, so limit that to 6 ounces per week.

- If you eat fish and shellfish from local waters, check with your health department for warnings about toxin-containing fish that should be avoided. If no information is available, limit yourself to 6 ounces per week and eat no other seafood that week, or avoid local seafood altogether.

Chapter Four

Preventing Infections

Infections are one of the main causes of birth defects and pregnancy complications. Fortunately, most of the infections that harm mothers and babies can be prevented or treated, reducing the risk of many infection-related health problems.

The best way to protect yourself and your baby from infections is to avoid getting them in the first place. There are several ways to do this:

- Shield yourself from infections that are spread by coughing, sneezing, and physical contact with germs by (when possible) staying away from children and adults who are sick and by not sharing eating utensils or toothbrushes.

- Steer clear of food-borne infections by handling and preparing foods safely—especially foods such as meat, eggs, and milk that have a higher risk of contamination by harmful bacteria. (For more information on food-borne infections, see chapter 3.)

- Avoid getting sexually transmitted infections by practicing safe sex. That means using a condom and not having sex with new partners, more than one partner, or an infected partner.

If you suspect you have any kind of infection—either because someone in your family has it, because you've eaten an unsafe food, or because you've noticed a suspicious symptom—call your provider right away and get it checked. Some infections clear up more easily if they are found and treated early.

If testing shows that you have an infection, your provider will advise you how to treat it. Some infections are easy to clear up with a medication that is considered safe for pregnant women. Other infection treatment is more complicated, requiring several drugs given at different times. With almost every infection, early diagnosis and treatment can increase a woman's chances of having a safe, successful pregnancy and a healthy baby.

Use the information in the following chart to protect yourself and your baby from infections:

Infection	Description	Possible symptoms	Prevention tips
Bacterial vaginosis	Vaginal infection that occurs when there's an overgrowth of bacteria in the vagina	Fishy-smelling white or gray vaginal discharge, burning during urination, vaginal itching, or no symptoms at all	Avoid douching; practice safe sex
Chickenpox	Viral infection that spreads through coughing, sneezing, and physical contact; can cause birth defects	Itchy, blistery rash and fever	Have a chickenpox (varicella) vaccination at least one month before getting pregnant if you're not already immune; the vaccine isn't recommended during pregnancy, so if you aren't immune, avoid anyone who has chickenpox or shingles, a condition caused by the same virus
Common cold	Viral infection that spreads through coughing, sneezing, and contact with an infected person; won't hurt you or your baby, but can be annoying	Runny nose, sore throat, stuffy head, cough, congestion	As much as possible, stay away from people with colds; wash your hands often, and don't share eating utensils
Cytomega-lovirus infection	Viral infection that's common during childhood; most adults are immune because they had it as children, but some are not; can cause intellectual disabilities in baby	Flulike symptoms such as fever, sore throat, swollen glands; or no symptoms	Avoid contact with children who may have it; if you are around sick children, wash your hands often and don't share eating utensils

Infection	Description	Possible symptoms	Prevention tips
Flu (influenza)	Viral infection that causes respiratory illness that can become severe or even life-threatening in pregnant women; can cause early birth	High fever, headache, fatigue, coughing, sore throat, runny nose, muscle aches, nausea, vomiting, diarrhea	Avoid contact with anyone who has the flu—the virus spreads in the air and by touch; have a flu shot during flu season (October/November through March/April in North America)
Group A strep infection	Bacterial infection that can cause strep throat, high fever	Sore throat, swollen glands, fever, sunburn-like rash on trunk and limbs	Avoid contact with anyone who may have it; if you are around sick people, wash your hands often and don't share eating utensils
Group B strep infection	Infection caused by bacteria found in the vagina and rectum of 25 percent of healthy women; can pass from mother to baby during vaginal birth; can cause blood infection in baby, pneumonia in mother	None	Get tested for it at 35 to 37 weeks of pregnancy; if you test positive, talk to your provider about antibiotic treatment during labor and birth to protect baby from infection
Parvovirus B19 infection (also called fifth disease)	Viral infection that's common during childhood; most adults are immune because they had it as children, but some are not; can cause miscarriage, anemia	In adults: flulike symptoms, joint pain, sometimes a red face rash; in children: fever, headache, sore throat, and a facial rash that looks like a slapped cheek	Avoid contact with children who might have it; if you are around sick children, wash your hands often after handling tissues and diapers and don't share eating utensils; if you've been exposed, call your provider right away
Pertussis (whooping cough)	Highly contagious respiratory illness; inhaling can make a "whooping" sound. In babies (especially newborns who have not yet received their vaccinations) and children, the disease can be very serious or even fatal	Runny nose, low-grade fever, cough; violent coughing fits can make it difficult to breathe	Have a Tdap booster shot before becoming pregnant, during pregnancy (preferably after 20 weeks), or immediately postpartum; encourage everyone who comes in contact with your newborn, such as dad, grandparents, siblings, and caregivers, to have their Tdap boosters also

Infection	Description	Possible symptoms	Prevention tips
Rubella (German measles)	Viral infection that can cause birth defects	Fever, swollen glands, facial rash, headache, flulike symptoms	Have a rubella vaccine at least one month before getting pregnant if you are not already immune; the vaccine isn't recommended during pregnancy, so if you aren't immune, avoid anyone who has rubella
Tuberculosis (TB)	Bacterial infection of the lungs that can spread to the mother's brain, kidneys, or spine; can cause low-birthweight baby	Coughing (sometimes with bloody discharge), chest pain, fatigue, fever, weight loss	Avoid contact with an infected person; TB spreads by touch or in the air
Urinary tract infection (UTI)	Bacterial infection of the urinary tract; can cause kidney infection and preterm birth	Pain and burning while urinating, frequent need to urinate, abdominal pain, fever	Urinate after sex, drink plenty of water, wipe from front to back after bowel movements
Yeast infection	Overgrowth of yeast found in the vagina; occurs more commonly in pregnant women	Itching, burning, and redness in the vaginal area; sometimes a cheesy white discharge	Avoid tight-fitting synthetic underwear that prevents air circulation in vaginal area; wipe from front to back after bowel movements; avoid use of douches, sprays, and other scented chemicals in vaginal area

IN DEPTH

Recognizing and Avoiding Sexually Transmitted Infections

See page 246

Chapter Five

Move Your Body

If you're like many women, you know you should exercise.

But . . .

You have a long list of excuses. You don't have time. You're too tired. You can't afford to join a gym. You get out of breath trying to jog. You don't know what to wear. You feel self-conscious.

So instead of exercising, you put your feet up and watch TV.

It's understandable. Life is busy, and it's hard to find the time and energy for exercise. But even if you've never managed to make exercise a routine, it's worthwhile to try again now that you're pregnant. Why? Because most women find that once they push past all those excuses and start to get active, great things happen. They begin to feel stronger, more toned, and more energetic. Fueled by good feelings, they keep moving, and the benefits of exercise start to multiply.

Like so many other healthy habits, exercise is great for pregnant women and their babies. And unless you have certain complications (see box on page 61), moderate exercise is perfectly safe when you're pregnant.

There are many reasons to exercise during pregnancy. It lowers the risk of a bunch of pregnancy complications, including gestational diabetes, high blood pressure, and deep vein thrombosis (a blood clot in the leg).

Exercise can also help reduce or relieve some of the discomforts of pregnancy, including backaches, constipation, bloating, swelling, and varicose veins.

And because it builds stamina and strengthens your muscles, exercise can help you be better prepared for labor and childbirth and bounce back to your preconception weight and fitness level after you give birth.

Activity provides emotional benefits as well. When you exercise, your body produces brain chemicals that boost your mood. Exercise can give you energy and help improve the way you feel about your growing, changing body. It can also help you sleep better and keep your weight in check.

YOU DON'T HAVE TO BE FIT TO EXERCISE

Every woman who is cleared for exercise by her provider can get out and move, even if she's never exercised before, is overweight, or even is obese.

You don't have to join a gym or run marathons—just taking a walk is beneficial. In fact, walking is one of the best activities for pregnant women. It's simple, inexpensive, and requires no training or special equipment other than a pair of supportive shoes. You can walk alone or with friends, in a city neighborhood or a leafy park, early in the morning, during your lunch break, or in the evening after dinner.

Not only is activity safe during pregnancy, but it's actually quite good for moms and babies in a variety of ways.

If you've never exercised before, don't worry—it's easier and more enjoyable than you may realize to add activity to your life.

What's 30 Minutes?

Women with low-risk pregnancies are advised to exercise *for at least 30 minutes a day most days of the week*—the same as nonpregnant women.

Thirty minutes may sound like a lot, especially if you haven't exercised much in the past. But remember, it's a goal that you can work toward, not something you have to go out and do on your first day.

Don't focus too much on what you *should* be doing. Instead, think about what you *can* do. Start small, and increase your exercise time gradually. Break your activity into chunks of 10 or 15 minutes, rather than waiting until you have an entire half hour free. Push yourself a bit, but not too much—you want to get something out of your activity, but you don't want to be so tired and sore the next day that you won't feel like moving. And if you miss a few days, just get back on track—don't try to jam a week's worth of exercise into one afternoon.

Enjoyment is one of the best motivators—so try to find ways to *have fun* while you exercise. Here are some strategies that might work for you:

- Choose activities you like.
- Exercise with friends or your partner.
- Alternate your activities to ward off boredom.
- Listen to your favorite music while you work out.
- Walk in new and interesting places, such as beautiful parks or historical neighborhoods.
- Go to the mall and window-shop while you walk.
- Reward yourself with little presents—a bouquet of flowers, for example—when you reach progress goals.

TURN YOUR WALK INTO A WORKOUT

Anytime you get out and go for a walk it's good for your body. But pushing things up a notch—in a way that's safe for you and your baby—can be even better. A brisk walk provides more benefits than a slow stroll, and a longer walk does more than a short one.

Q: *What kind of shoe is best for walking?*

A: *The best choice is a shoe with a flexible sole, good arch support, and cushioning in the heel. Sporting goods stores and many shoe stores sell sneakers specifically designed for walking. An inexpensive pair is fine as long as it supports and cushions your foot. Shoes made for other sports may not be comfortable for long walks—for example, walking in running shoes may cause soreness in your shins. Let your feet be your guide, and go with whatever shoes feel best.*

Q: *Does exercise increase risk of miscarriage, preterm labor, or birth defects?*

A: *No. In fact, studies have found that when healthy women having a low-risk pregnancy exercise moderately, their risk of preterm birth goes down.*

If walking is your exercise of choice, absolutely start where you feel comfortable, even if it's short and slow. But then, over time, consider pumping up your walking workouts.

It's fine to intensify your walking gradually—in fact, that's the best way, because if you do too much too soon, you end up with sore muscles and not much interest in getting out there the next day.

Begin with as little as five minutes of easy walking once a day. Then kick it up a bit each week as you become fitter and better able to tolerate the challenges of your activity. There are three ways to do this:

1. Walk longer. Each week, add five minutes to your daily total, aiming for an eventual goal of at least 30 minutes a day.

2. Walk faster. When you're ready, start focusing on going a little faster. Begin with short bursts of speed mixed with regular walking—for example, speed up for one minute, then walk at your normal pace for four minutes, and repeat. This is called interval training. If you walk in a neighborhood, try increasing your pace in front of every third or fourth house. Over time, lengthen your speedy intervals until you're going faster for your entire walk. (Even then, though, begin your walk with a five-minute warm-up walk at a comfortable pace to give your heart and muscles time to prepare for a higher-intensity walk.)

3. Walk more frequently. When you've topped out at your best speed and time, you can boost your intensity by adding some additional walks to your weekly routine. For example, if you usually do a half hour every morning, add an additional 10-minute walk after dinner one or two nights a week. Or add in a long walk on the weekend—gather up some friends, go to a park, and walk off the week's stresses.

Remember, your goal is to exercise *moderately*. If you can't pass the "talk test"—being able to talk easily while you walk—slow down. Your goal is to exercise at a healthy pace, not to push yourself so hard that it becomes unsafe for you or your baby.

THE BEST EXERCISES FOR YOU

The best prenatal activities are those that allow you to work your heart and muscles in a way that's safe for you and your baby. Walking fits the bill perfectly, but there are other great options as well.

Swimming Pregnant women tend to enjoy swimming because the water supports their weight and keeps them cool. Using your muscles to push through the resistance of the water helps improve circulation and strengthen your muscles and your heart. If you like to swim, opt for laps in the pool or a water aerobics class designed for pregnant women.

Gym machines You may like using a treadmill, a stationary or recumbent bicycle, or an elliptical trainer. Each provides an excellent aerobic workout. Before hopping on any new piece of exercise equipment, be sure to ask for instructions so you can use it safely.

Prenatal fitness classes Prenatal fitness classes offer another great exercise alternative (if they are taught by a certified instructor with training in pregnancy fitness). They provide a workout and a chance to meet and socialize with other pregnant women. Look for prenatal fitness classes at your local Y, health club, hospital, or community education department, or ask your provider for a recommendation. Be sure to choose a class that is right for your fitness level. If a workout seems too difficult, adjust your pace or ask the instructor to show you how to modify the routine.

Prenatal yoga These popular classes mix meditative work and breathing exercises with poses that stretch, strengthen, and relax your body. There are many styles of yoga; most commonly, prenatal classes teach hatha yoga (a gentle type of yoga that emphasizes posture and breathing), with certain poses modified in a way that's safe for pregnant women. The relaxation training you learn in a yoga class can come in handy during labor and delivery. The downside of prenatal yoga is that it doesn't give your heart and lungs the kind of aerobic workout that you'd get from a brisk walk. If you have time, do both, because they're each good for you, but in different ways.

Home workouts If you prefer to exercise at home, you might like to use a prenatal exercise DVD that guides you through a workout. Choose one that matches your fitness level. Your public library may have prenatal exercise DVDs available for borrowing, allowing you to sample different approaches.

Strength training If you did strength training before pregnancy, you can keep doing it (with your provider's okay). If done correctly, strength training can be safe during a healthy, low-risk pregnancy. To be cautious, increase repetitions and decrease the amount of weight you lift. Be sure you're not straining or holding your breath as you train, and avoid lifting weights above your head, which can strain your back. As you gain weight and your center of gravity shifts, your posture changes, so it's best to work with an experienced spotter or trainer who can ensure that you're lifting properly and safely.

Personal training For an individualized approach, give personal training a try. Personal trainers—trained and certified fitness professionals—often work independently or at gyms and fitness centers. Although they can be expensive, personal trainers are helpful because they design an exercise program personalized to your particular fitness level and goals. They also teach you how to

Q: *How hard should I exercise?*

A: *During pregnancy, the best pace is brisk but moderate—intense enough to give you a benefit, but not hard enough to wipe you out or limit the oxygen your baby receives from your blood. To determine whether you're pushing too hard, take the talk test: if you're too winded to hold a conversation while you're exercising, ease up a bit.*

exercise safely and effectively. You can meet with a trainer on a weekly basis to have guidance during your workout, or you can schedule just one or two meetings to kick-start your exercise program.

Higher-intensity workouts If you already exercise, higher-intensity sports such as jogging, running, and racket sports may be safe for you to continue doing. Check with your provider.

Kegels No matter what your fitness level, you can benefit from doing Kegel exercises, which are named after the doctor who first recommended them. They strengthen the muscles of your pelvic floor, rectum, vagina, urethra, and pelvis. Working these muscles during pregnancy will help you as you push during labor, aid in a quick recovery after you give birth, and help you control your bladder, which may leak a bit during and after pregnancy.

IN DEPTH

Exercise Guidelines for Pregnant Athletes

See page 248

To do a Kegel, simply squeeze the muscles that you use to stop a stream of urine. Try to keep your other muscles, such as your abdominals, relaxed. Hold the squeeze tight for a count of three; then relax for a count of three. Repeat 10 to 15 times, three times a day. Kegels can be done while standing, lying down, sitting, or even driving—some women make it a point to do a Kegel exercise whenever they're at a red light.

ACTIVITIES TO AVOID

Although exercise is generally safe during pregnancy, some types should be avoided for safety's sake. Generally it's best to stay away from any activity that puts you at risk for *falling, being injured,* or *getting too little oxygen.*

Falling becomes more of a concern as your belly grows and your center of gravity shifts. Because of the added weight at the front of your body, you may become less steady on your feet. Falling can injure you and your baby. That's why it's best to avoid activities done on unstable ground where you're more likely to trip, such as hiking on terrain with lots of loose stones and exposed roots.

You can also prevent dangerous falls by choosing not to do gymnastics or go skating, downhill skiing, waterskiing, or horseback riding. Riding a bike can become unsafe later in your pregnancy, when your balance is less steady.

Q: *Does exercise make labor and childbirth easier?*

A: *No matter how fit you are, giving birth is painful. However, studies suggest that women who exercise during pregnancy may be better equipped to deal with the pain of childbirth, and they may have more stamina to withstand labor. In addition, some women who do prenatal yoga find that meditative breathing exercises practiced in the yoga studio help them stay relaxed in the delivery room.*

Your risk of injury goes up if you do high-impact exercise that calls for bouncy, jerky movements, such as a high-impact aerobics class. The hormones of pregnancy allow your muscles and joint ligaments to relax in order to make extra room for your growing baby, but relaxed joints are more prone to injury during high-impact activity.

Getting hit in the abdominal area by a ball or a person is unsafe during pregnancy, so sit out contact sports such as soccer and kickboxing.

Altitude can impact your baby's ability to get enough oxygen. Avoid high-altitude (over 6,000 feet) activities such as mountain climbing. Going low can be as problematic as going high: scuba diving can put unacceptable pressure on your baby's body and create dangerous gas bubbles in your baby's blood.

EXERCISING RIGHT

Exercising during pregnancy is safe—as long as you keep these tips in mind:

Stay cool Elevating your body temperature even a couple of degrees isn't good for your baby, especially in early pregnancy. When you're exercising outdoors, wear easy-to-remove layers, and plan your outings for the coolest times of day.

Opt for an indoor activity when heat and humidity are high. Indoors, wear loose clothes that allow air circulation, and use a fan or air-conditioning to keep the room temperature down. Stay out of steam rooms, hot tubs, and saunas; don't do "hot yoga"; and skip your workout if you have a fever.

Keep the oxygen flowing You and your baby both need a steady supply of oxygen, so take a few simple steps to ensure a healthy flow. Keep your exercise at a moderate level—work hard enough that you feel your heart rate and your breathing rate increase, but not so hard that you have trouble talking.

Slow down or take a break if you're feeling out of breath or too tuckered to talk. If you strength-train, be sure not to hold your breath while lifting.

Drink water Have some water before, during, and after exercising. You may need to use the restroom more often than you used to, so plan accordingly.

Stay fueled You won't have much energy if you work out on an empty stomach. If your tank needs some fuel, choose a healthy snack of about 300 calories that contains high-quality protein and a whole-grain food—for example, peanut butter on whole-wheat toast, fruit and yogurt, cheese and crackers, or beans and rice.

If you're going to be exercising for a while, take along an easy-to-eat snack such as trail mix made with nuts, dried fruit, and toasted oat cereal. Keep an eye on your weight, and if you're not gaining enough on a week-by-week basis, boost your portion sizes a bit.

Support yourself Wear an exercise bra that keeps your breasts from bouncing uncomfortably.

Stay off your back After your first trimester, skip any moves that require you to lie flat on your back. The weight of your belly may interfere with blood circulation in the major blood vessels in your body's core, which could limit blood flow to your baby.

When to Stop Exercising

Immediately stop exercising and call your provider if any of the following occur:

- *Abdominal pain*
- *Blurred vision*
- *Calf pain or swelling*
- *Chest pain*
- *Contractions*
- *Decreased fetal movement*
- *Dizziness*
- *Headache*
- *Lightheadedness*
- *Unexplained shortness of breath*
- *Vaginal bleeding or fluid leakage*

Practice outdoor safety If you exercise outdoors, be smart about where and when you walk or jog. Always carry identification and a charged cell phone, be aware of your surroundings at all times, wear reflective clothing if you're out at night, and pay close attention to cars, bicycles, dogs, and other pedestrians. To stay alert to traffic and other dangers, leave your earbuds off or keep the volume down.

Listen to your body If you feel unexpectedly tired or sluggish, or if you think an exercise or yoga pose isn't right for you, stop. You know your body better than anyone else does.

Q: *Can I do sit-ups while I'm pregnant?*

A: *In moderation, sit-ups are fine during the first trimester, but avoid any exercises that require you to lie flat on your back during the second and third trimesters. To tone your abdominal muscles, kneel down on your hands and knees and pull your abs in; hold, then release. If you're starting to think too much about doing sit-ups, though, take a step back and consider your motivation. Some women respond to the growth of their baby bump by adding lots and lots of sit-ups to their exercise regimen. Although it's good to maintain abdominal strength during pregnancy, it's best not to go overboard.*

Q: *While we're on the topic of physical activity—is it safe to have sex while I'm pregnant?*

A: *It's fine for most women. Your provider may recommend abstinence if you have certain complications, such as placenta previa, amniotic fluid leakage, an elevated risk of preterm birth or miscarriage, or unexplained vaginal discharge, bleeding, or cramping.*

You may find that sex is actually more enjoyable during pregnancy, because you don't have to deal with birth control. However, it's important to stay free of STIs, because they can raise the risk of miscarriage, preterm delivery, stillbirth, and birth defects. To avoid getting an STI, have sex with only one person—a person who doesn't have an STI and who doesn't have any other sex partners. If you suspect that your partner has an STI, use a condom or, even better, don't have sex until you're both tested and treated. This is especially important for a woman who has a new sex partner.

Chapter Six

Weighing Your Options

Now it's time to talk about most pregnant women's *least* favorite topic: weight.

Weight is a big source of concern—and worry—during pregnancy. Underweight women may struggle to gain enough. Overweight women may worry about gaining too much. Rare is the woman who starts her pregnancy at the perfect weight, jumps happily onto the scale at every prenatal appointment, and hits her weight-gain bull's-eye in the last week of her pregnancy.

It can be hard for any woman to embrace the idea of being told to put on 20, 30, or even 40 pounds. But gaining the right amount of weight while you're pregnant is worth the effort. Weight gain during pregnancy isn't about looks; it's a medical issue.

Gaining the just-right amount of weight—not too much, not too little—helps ensure that both you and your baby get the energy and nutrients necessary to support all of the amazing changes going on inside you. It also boosts your odds of having an uncomplicated pregnancy, a routine labor and childbirth, and a healthy, full-term baby.

If you gain more weight than what's recommended, a few risk factors start to rise. Your chance of developing gestational diabetes goes up, for example, as does the likelihood that you will hold on to the extra weight after your baby is born. Women who are very overweight at delivery—either because they gained more than advised or because they began their pregnancy obese—are more likely to need a c-section, in part because their babies are often bigger than average.

Gaining too little weight has disadvantages, too. Because you're less likely to get enough nutrients when you gain less than recommended, your baby may develop slowly—a condition known as fetal growth restriction—which can lead to health problems after birth and beyond. There's also a higher chance of your baby being born early or with a low birthweight and having trouble breathing or keeping blood sugar at a safe level.

The good news is that even though it may be a bit of a struggle to gain the optimal amount of weight, it is something you have some control over. There are many parts of pregnancy you *can't* control—your genetics, for example. But you *can* make choices starting now and throughout your entire pregnancy that help you meet your weight-gain goals.

Even if you're starting your pregnancy over or under your ideal weight, you can take steps to make your pregnancy as healthy as it can be.

HOW MUCH WEIGHT SHOULD YOU GAIN?

Based on your health and your preconception weight, your provider arrives at a weight-gain recommendation that's best for you. This is based on your body mass index, or BMI, which is calculated using your height and weight. Your preconception BMI determines if you are underweight (BMI under 18.5), normal weight (BMI 18.5 to 24.9), overweight (BMI 25 to 29.9), or obese (BMI over 30). You can calculate your BMI at www.nhlbisupport.com/bmi/ or use the chart on page 249 of the "In Depth" section.

Generally, the following weight guidelines apply for women carrying a single baby:

Preconception weight	Recommended weight gain during pregnancy
Underweight	28 to 40 pounds
Normal weight	25 to 35 pounds
Overweight	15 to 25 pounds
Obese	11 to 20 pounds

> **Q:** *I hate getting weighed at my provider's office. Can't I just skip it?*
>
> **A:** *Unfortunately, you can't. As irritating as it might be, getting weighed is necessary, because it gives your provider information that helps guide the course of your prenatal care.*
>
> *Weighing in can be one of the most stressful parts of a prenatal visit. When your provider checks your weight and writes it down in your chart, you may feel you're being judged—as if your efforts at being healthy during pregnancy all come down to a single number, like the grade on a test. Many women link the numbers on the scale with self-esteem and self-worth. You might feel good when you see certain numbers and bad when you see others— it's a common habit for women who have struggled with their weight.*
>
> *If you'd rather not know the number on the scale, ask your provider not to tell you, simply to write it down without comment.*

Weight-gain recommendations go up for mothers carrying multiples. The general guidelines for twins are 37 to 54 pounds (normal-weight women), 31 to 50 pounds (overweight women), and 25 to 42 pounds (obese women). If you are underweight and expecting twins, or are pregnant with triplets or more, your provider will help you figure out how much to gain.

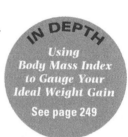

IN DEPTH

Using
Body Mass Index
to Gauge Your
Ideal Weight Gain

See page 249

REACHING YOUR WEIGHT GOAL

Once you know your recommended weight-gain target, you can start thinking about how much and what kinds of food you need to eat on a daily basis in order to stay on track with your goal.

One way to do this is to count calories. If this is the right strategy for you, your provider can help you figure out a daily calorie goal that's based on several factors, including your height, preconception weight, activity level, muscle mass, frame size, and general health. Then you can use food labels to figure out how much to eat.

An easier way is just to keep your eye on the scale. If you're gaining the right amount of weight, you're probably eating enough. If you're gaining too much or too little, look at how much and the kinds of food you're eating.

Either way—whether by counting calories or by monitoring the scale—you can make some changes in what and how much you eat so your weight gain starts to track more closely to these recommendations:

- *First trimester (13 weeks).* Gain a total of 2 to 4 pounds. Note, though, that some women gain nothing, especially if they have morning sickness. As long as you're not underweight to start with, it's okay if you don't gain during early pregnancy.

- *Second and third trimesters.* Gain about 1 pound a week if you start pregnancy in the normal-weight range. Target gains are higher if you're underweight and lower if you're overweight or obese. Your provider can work with you to calculate your own personal weekly and monthly weight-gain goals.

Keep in mind that these weekly targets are averages. It's normal to have occasional dips and spurts: you may gain nothing for two weeks and then add several pounds in one week. As long as your weight sticks with the basic trajectory of healthy gain over the course of your pregnancy, you are on target.

If you need help managing your weight, ask your provider about referring you to a nutritionist. Many prenatal practices and clinics have nutritionists on staff, and visits with them are often covered by health insurance.

DO THE MATH: CALCULATING YOUR DAILY CALORIE NEEDS

Here's an example of how daily calorie needs for a normal-weight or overweight woman might be calculated. (Different guidelines may apply to underweight and obese women. If you fall into one of those groups, consult your provider.)

Start with your preconception calorie needs:

- Nonpregnant women who are sedentary (get no exercise beyond the light physical activity associated with day-to-day life) need roughly 1,800 to 2,000 calories daily.

- Nonpregnant women who are moderately active (walking about 1½ to 3 miles per day at 3 to 4 miles per hour, or equivalent exertion, in addition to the light physical activity associated with day-to-day life) need roughly 2,000 to 2,200 calories daily.

- Nonpregnant women who are active (walking more than 3 miles per day at 3 to 4 miles per hour, or equivalent exertion, in addition to the light physical activity associated with typical day-to-day life) need roughly 2,200 to 2,400 calories daily.

Once the preconception calorie range is determined, it can be adjusted in this way to take into account the additional calories necessary during pregnancy:

- **First trimester.** The number of calories you consumed before you conceived should be enough during the first 14 weeks or so of pregnancy, so your daily calorie target stays the same.

- **Second and third trimesters.** During the remainder of your pregnancy, you need an additional 300 calories per day to sustain a healthy pregnancy.

Using these standard numbers, calorie recommendations look like this:

Approximate Daily Calorie Targets During Pregnancy (For normal-weight and overweight women)			
	Sedentary	Moderately Active	Active
First trimester	1,800 to 2,000 calories	2,000 to 2,200 calories	2,200 to 2,400 calories
Second and third trimesters	2,100 to 2,300	2,300 to 2,500	2,500 to 2,700

Remember, these are just *guidelines*, and they're targeted at women with a preconception BMI between 18.5 and 29.9. Your calorie count may vary.

Q: *At what weights are newborns considered very small or very big?*

A: *Generally, a low-birthweight baby weighs less than 5.5 pounds (2,500 grams) and a macrosomic (large-birthweight) baby weighs over 8.8 pounds (4,000 grams).*

Smart Snacks

During the second and third trimesters, you need about 300 extra calories a day. It may be tempting to splurge on your favorite junk foods, but it's best to skip the cupcakes and candy bars and use those extra calories more wisely.

Healthy snacks provide nutrients you need and keep you satisfied between meals. But they don't have to be boring—there are lots of delicious ways to snack healthfully. Here are some suggestions for nutritious snacks that weigh in at approximately 200 to 300 calories.

- *1 cup fat-free vanilla yogurt and a medium banana*

- *1 slice whole-wheat toast with 2 tablespoons peanut butter*

- *1 cup raisin bran cereal and 1 cup skim milk*

- *1 corn tortilla stuffed with ½ cup black beans, some shredded lettuce, ½ cup chopped tomato, and 2 tablespoons shredded cheddar*

- *1 cup chili with beans*

- *1 cup nonfat cottage cheese with 1 cup fresh strawberries*

- *1 cup low-sodium vegetable or split-pea soup with five sesame crackers*

- *1 ounce baked tortilla chips with ¼ cup guacamole and ¼ cup fresh tomato salsa*

- *A toasted cheese and tomato sandwich made with two slices whole-wheat bread, 1 slice cheese, and sliced tomato*

- *1 medium apple and 1 cup cooked oatmeal made with ½ cup skim milk*

- *Spinach salad made with 2 cups fresh spinach, 1 chopped hard-boiled egg, ½ cup fresh mushrooms, and 2 tablespoons olive oil vinaigrette*

- *½ cup vanilla pudding (made with milk) topped with ½ cup blueberries*

- *2 scrambled eggs, 1 slice whole-wheat toast, and ½ cup orange juice*

- *A pizza made with 1 whole-grain English muffin, 1 tablespoon spaghetti sauce, and 2 tablespoons shredded mozzarella*

- *An omelet made with 2 eggs, ½ cup broccoli, and 2 tablespoons shredded cheddar*

Where Does the Weight Gain Go?

A gain of 28½ to 30½ pounds—in the middle range for a normal-weight woman—gets distributed something like this:

Baby	6 to 8 pounds
Placenta	1½ pounds
Amniotic fluid	2 pounds
Uterus growth	2 pounds
Breast growth	2 pounds
Your body's blood and other fluids	8 pounds
Your body's protein and fat	7 pounds

AIM FOR GOOD GAIN

Although it's not okay to diet during pregnancy, it's good to adjust your daily calorie intake to meet the healthy targets you and your provider have set. It's crucial to maintain a well-balanced diet and to eat foods from every food group. No-carb or no-fat dieting is not good for you or your baby.

The best way to trim excess calories is to cut back on sugary desserts, high-fat junk food, unhealthy saturated fats, and other so-called empty calories—those that have few or no nutrients. An excellent place to start is to replace sugary soft drinks such as soda, sweetened ice tea, sports drinks, and fruit punches with water, seltzer, or other unsweetened beverages. This switch alone can save you a huge number of calories if you're a big soda drinker. Consider this: a single 12-ounce can of cola has about 140 calories, almost 10 teaspoons of sugar, and absolutely no nutrients.

IN DEPTH

Pregnancy After Weight-Loss Surgery

See page 251

You can also choose lower-fat versions of nutritious foods such as milk. Switching from whole milk to fat-free saves you up to 60 calories a cup without giving up any calcium or vitamin D. If you use cream in your coffee, choosing skim milk instead saves you about 90 calories in a 2-tablespoon serving size.

Keep a closer eye on portion sizes, too—refer to the daily food group listings in chapter 3 for portion-size specifics. Try measuring your food rather than estimating serving sizes. You might be surprised to see that the bowl of cereal you thought was one serving's worth is actually two or even three. And consider keeping a food diary in which you record everything you eat for a couple of days—it may help you see where your excess calories are coming from.

If you are gaining too much too fast, don't beat yourself up. Instead of dwelling on it, start cutting out empty calories and look forward instead of back.

Give Your Plate a Makeover

Make these changes to cut down on empty calories without losing any nutrients:

Instead of:	Try this:
Deep-fried meat	Baked, broiled, stir-fried, or poached meat
Fatty meat and poultry	Lean meat with visible fat cut off and skin removed
Full-fat mayonnaise, cheese, sour cream, and salad dressings	Low-fat or nonfat versions; or simply use half of what you ordinarily use
Cream sauces or butter on vegetables	A squirt of fresh lemon and a sprinkle of fresh or dried herbs
Refried beans	Black beans
A full-size chocolate bar	A small square of decadent dark chocolate
Canned fruit packed in sugary syrup	Fresh fruit, or canned fruit packed in its own juice
Creamy pasta sauce	Tomato-based pasta sauce
Tuna packed in oil	Tuna packed in water
Sugary breakfast cereals	Unsweetened breakfast cereals with sliced banana or berries
High-fat snacks such as potato chips	Unbuttered popcorn flavored with a sprinkle of parmesan cheese
Full-fat ice cream	Reduced-fat ice cream, frozen yogurt, ice milk, sorbet, or sherbet
Medium, large, or supersize servings in a restaurant	Small or kid's-size servings

Q: *If I'm gaining too much weight too fast, can exercise help slow it down?*

A: *Exercise does use up calories—but the burn is somewhat modest, so you can't expect an afternoon walk to make up for a day of overeating. Walking briskly for 30 minutes is good for you in so many ways, but it burns only about 130 calories or so. Exercise complements a healthy diet, but it's no substitute for smart eating.*

IN DEPTH

Pregnancy Advice for Obese Women

See page 252

Q: *I started my pregnancy overweight. Can I go on a low-calorie diet now and try not to gain any weight at all?*

A: *Unless you're quite obese, dieting is risky during pregnancy. If your body doesn't get the energy (calories) it requires for you and your baby from the food you eat, it uses your body fat for energy. This fat burn produces chemicals called ketones, which are not good for your baby's brain.*

PERSONALIZE A PLAN FOR WEIGHT GAIN

You step on the scale at your provider's office and are surprised to see that the number hasn't changed much since your last visit. Your provider suggests that you add extra calories to your diet—but not just any calories. The best strategy is to eat more nutritious foods that are good for you and your baby. That way, the extra food you eat delivers important nutrients and not just empty calories.

IN DEPTH

Pregnancy Advice for Underweight Women

See page 253

For ideas on what kinds of foods to add to your diet, go back to the food group goals in chapter 3 and compare them to your daily diet. Look for differences between what's recommended and what's on your plate. Are you getting enough dairy? Fruit? Is a fear of carbohydrates keeping you from eating bread?

Once you figure out which foods you can use more of, make a plan. If you're short on protein and carbohydrates, for example, add in a turkey sandwich for an afternoon snack. If you're not getting enough dairy and fruit, pull out the blender to whip up breakfast smoothies made with yogurt and bananas, strawberries, blueberries, or black cherries. If you're short on vegetables and healthy fats, dip carrots, peppers, and celery sticks into hummus or guacamole.

Here are some other ways to add healthy, nutritious calories to your daily menu:

- Add in healthy snacks midmorning, midafternoon, or two hours before bedtime.
- Increase portion sizes of nutritious foods. If you're not hungry enough for bigger portions, try having an additional meal in the middle of the afternoon.
- Snack on almonds, peanuts, hazelnuts, pecans, walnuts, cashews, or other nuts, which are dense in calories. In addition to beneficial fats, nuts contain an array of vitamins and minerals, including folate, iron, fiber, and calcium. Nuts also taste good mixed into salads and granola.
- Sprinkle seeds onto salads and entrees, or snack on them out of hand. Like nuts, seeds such as pumpkin, sesame, and sunflower are rich in nutrients and calories.
- Stir wheat germ into yogurt or breakfast cereal. It's high in folate and fiber as well as calories.
- Spread nut butters (peanut, almond, cashew) on whole-grain bread, English muffins, or bagels for a fast, easy snack.
- Consider switching from low-fat to full-fat foods such as salad dressings, dairy foods, and cheese.
- Drizzle some extra olive oil on your salads. This heart-healthy oil is a good source of omega-3 fatty acids, which are good for your heart and your baby's growing brain.
- Choose fatty, higher-calorie fish such as salmon rather than leaner, lower-fat fish such as cod.
- Carry a calorie-rich trail mix with you and nibble on it when you feel hungry. Buy it premade or make your own by combining nuts, dried fruit, pretzels, flaked coconut, chocolate chips, seeds, toasted oats, dry cereal, yogurt-covered raisins, and whatever else you might enjoy.
- Add avocado to your diet—toss it into salads, slice it onto sandwiches, and dip crackers and veggies into guacamole. The monounsaturated fat in avocado adds calories and omega-3 fatty acids to your diet.
- When heating up condensed soup (such as tomato), stir in milk rather than water.

Chapter Seven

If Things Get Uncomfortable

Being pregnant is a wonderful experience. But let's face it: pregnancy can also be pretty uncomfortable. It's the only time in your adult life when it's considered completely normal to pee when you laugh, have crazy mood swings, pass gas on a regular basis, get excited when you have a normal bowel movement, throw up even though you aren't sick, grow hair in odd places, eat crackers in bed, take naps in the middle of the day, and have nosebleeds for no reason.

Much of the blame for these bothersome symptoms can be pinned on the hormones that rule pregnancy. These hormones make it possible for you to get pregnant, carry your baby for three trimesters, and give birth. They relax muscles and ligaments so your baby has room to grow and then emerge.

Unfortunately, hormones also have some not-so-desirable effects on your pregnant body, such as loosening the muscles that hold urine in your bladder and food in your stomach.

Carrying all that weight around your middle also contributes to some of the discomforts of pregnancy. Your growing baby can press on your internal organs, slow down the circulation of your blood, make your back ache, and send you to the bathroom so often that you may feel you spend more time there than in any other room in your home.

> *While you throw up, belch, itch, toss and turn, worry, ache, pant, and waddle, your baby is busy growing and developing in a safe and secure environment, oblivious to your discomforts.*

The good news about most of these symptoms is that, although they are annoying, they generally cause no harm to you or your baby. While you throw up, belch, itch, toss and turn, worry, ache, pant, and waddle, your baby is busy growing and developing in a safe and secure environment, oblivious to your discomforts.

But that doesn't mean you just have to accept the physical inconveniences of pregnancy. This chapter covers the most common discomforts of pregnancy and offers prevention and coping tips that should help you feel better and more comfortable.

HOW TO GET BETTER SLEEP

It's a pregnancy paradox: you're tired, but you can't sleep. Why in the world does this happen to some women?

During early pregnancy, changes in hormone levels can affect your ability to get to sleep, stay asleep, and wake up feeling refreshed. As your baby grows, you may have trouble finding a comfortable sleep position. Other pregnancy-related discomforts, such as heartburn, nasal congestion, and hemorrhoids, can keep you awake at night, as can stress and anxiety about becoming a mother. And having to get up once or twice (or more often) to go to the bathroom during the night certainly doesn't help.

Some days you may feel tired even when you get plenty of sleep. That's normal, especially in the first trimester, when your body is adjusting to pregnancy and your baby's body is experiencing tremendous change. Fatigue usually improves somewhat in the second trimester. Then in the third trimester it often comes back.

There are ways to get the ZZZs you crave. Try these sleep-boosting tips:

- *Schedule more time in bed.* It can be difficult to carve time out of a busy day, but if you can possibly manage it, try to go to bed earlier, set the morning alarm later, and plan daytime naps.

- **Relax before bed.** If you often find yourself lying in bed feeling stressed, try a new routine: spend 20 minutes or so before you retire doing something relaxing—listening to calming music, meditating, reading, taking a warm shower, or getting a backrub from your partner.

- **Cut back on liquids near bedtime.** Reducing or avoiding evening beverages may save you a trip to the bathroom during the night.

- **Create a sleepy atmosphere.** Pregnancy may change the way light, sound, and temperature affect your sleep. Make your bedroom sleep-friendly with room-darkening shades or eyeshades to block light, a white-noise machine or earplugs to block sound, and an air conditioner or heater so the temperature is just right for you.

- **Prop yourself with pillows.** Sleeping flat on your back can be uncomfortable while you're pregnant. It's also not recommended for your baby. After your first trimester, when you lie on your back the weight of your baby can press down on the major blood vessels that travel beneath your uterus. This pressure may interfere with your blood flow and with circulation of blood to your baby. Use pillows behind your back, between your knees, and under your belly to support a cozy side-sleeping position—preferably on your left side, which allows better circulation. Some women like using a large body pillow.

Q: *Some nights I wake up with a tight, painful cramp in my leg. What should I do?*

A: *First, don't worry. Leg cramps are common during pregnancy. Changes in blood flow, extra weight, and pressure on nerves and blood vessels in the legs can sometimes cause leg muscles to cramp and tighten. Leg cramps are most likely to happen at night during the second and third trimesters. When you get a cramp, stretch your leg by straightening it out heel first and wiggling (but not pointing) your toes. Then relax the muscle with massage, heat, a warm shower, or a walk. To help prevent leg cramps, drink plenty of water, stretch your calves before bed, exercise daily, and don't stand or sit in one position for long—get up and walk around every 30 minutes or so. Contact your provider if your leg cramps don't go away or are severe.*

- **Notice how exercise affects you.** Some women find that exercising close to bedtime keeps them awake; others find that a late-evening walk helps make them sleepy. Be mindful of what works for you.

- **Stay away from sleep remedies.** Don't take over-the-counter or prescription sleep medicines, herbal teas, melatonin, or any other sleep remedy without your provider's approval.

- **Mention fatigue to your provider.** Fatigue is a symptom of anemia and some other conditions that are common during pregnancy, so your provider may want to do a blood test if you're feeling especially fatigued.

CONSTIPATION SOLUTIONS

Few women make it through pregnancy without occasionally struggling to pass a bowel movement, putting up with constipation-related belly pain and cramping, having fewer than three bowel movements a week, or passing hard, small stools.

Why does it happen? Pregnancy hormones slow down the digestive system because they relax the smooth muscle around the bowels. Unfortunately, this slowing can contribute to constipation. It can get even worse as your pregnancy goes on and the weight of your growing baby presses down on your intestines.

High-Fiber Foods

Ready for more roughage? These foods are excellent sources of fiber:

- *Beans (black, lima, pinto, kidney, etc.)*
- *Lentils*
- *Baked potato with skin*
- *Fruits such as pears, apples, and berries*
- *Dried fruits such as raisins, apricots, and prunes (as well as prune juice)*
- *Vegetables*
- *Whole-grain pasta, bread, and bagels*
- *Whole-grain cereals such as raisin bran and bran flakes*
- *Oatmeal*
- *Nuts*

If you want to eat more fiber, adjust your diet gradually, adding a bit more each day. Boosting fiber intake too quickly can cause bloating and gas.

Q: *Why do I have to pee so often?*

A: *There are a few reasons for this. Your body contains more fluids during pregnancy, mainly because your blood volume increases by almost 50 percent. In addition, your bladder can be compressed by the uterus and hold less urine before it feels full. Finally, pregnancy hormones cause a relaxing of the muscles at the opening of your bladder. When these muscles relax, you need to urinate more often. You may also leak urine when you laugh, cough, sneeze, or exercise.*

To strengthen those muscles, do Kegel exercises by squeezing the muscles you use to stop the flow of urine and holding them for 10 seconds; repeat 10 to 20 times in a row at least three times a day. If frequent peeing interrupts your sleep, avoid drinking liquids right before bed.

Be sure to call your provider if you feel burning or pain while urinating, or if the urge to urinate continues after you empty your bladder. These can be symptoms of an infection in your bladder or urinary tract.

The iron in prenatal vitamins can also contribute to constipation, especially if your provider has advised you to take extra iron because of anemia.

If you're constipated, try these tips:

- **Drink up.** Getting enough water can help you pass stool more easily. An extra glass of water every few hours should help. Keep a bottle of water on your desk, in your car, by your bedside, or wherever you'll see it and remember to drink.

- **Fill up with fiber.** Eating more high-fiber foods is another way to add bulk to your stool and make it pass more quickly. To prevent belly cramps and gas, increase your fiber gradually, and drink plenty of water.

- **Listen when nature calls.** Avoid holding in a bowel movement when you feel the urge to go. Head straight for the bathroom.

- **Give yourself time.** Grab something to read, sit on the toilet, and give your bowels time to move. Straining can cause hemorrhoids.

- **Talk with your provider.** If these changes don't help, ask your provider about using a stool softener such as docusate sodium (brand name Colace). Avoid stimulant laxatives such as bisacodyl (brand name Dulcolax) unless recommended by your provider—they can produce strong, sudden bowel movements.

COOL THE HEARTBURN FIRE

Heartburn is another problem that strikes most pregnant women. For some, it's just a once-in-a-while inconvenience, but for others, it's a near-constant annoyance that gets worse as the weeks of pregnancy pass.

Also known as indigestion, reflux, or gastroesophageal reflux disease (GERD), heartburn occurs when stomach acid is pushed up into the esophagus, the tube that carries food from your throat to your stomach.

Pregnancy hormones can relax the flap that separates your esophagus from your stomach. This can allow the contents of your stomach—food and acidic digestive juices—to move back up into your esophagus and cause a burning feeling. Pressure on your stomach from your growing baby can also contribute to reflux. Not surprisingly, heartburn tends to worsen in the second and third trimesters, when your baby is getting bigger and taking up more space inside your body.

Heartburn causes a burning, painful, bloated feeling beneath your lower ribs and breastbone. You may also feel burning and discomfort in your neck and experience an unpleasant acid taste in the back of your mouth and throat.

To help relieve heartburn, try the following:

- **Graze.** Avoid big meals, because having a full stomach can make heartburn worse. Instead, eat smaller meals more frequently during the day.

- **Grab a spoon.** A few bites of plain nonfat yogurt can sometimes cool the burn.

> **Q:** *I have a lot of gas. What can I do to stop it?*
>
> **A:** *Passing gas is normal during pregnancy, but that doesn't make it any less embarrassing. It can also be uncomfortable—for example, when it's accompanied by bloating, burping, belching, and belly pain. To prevent gas, avoid large meals, eat slowly, and don't drink from straws, chew gum, or suck on hard candy, all of which can cause you to swallow air. Possible food culprits include beans and whole grains (especially if you recently increased your fiber intake), vegetables such as cabbage and broccoli, starchy foods such as pasta and potatoes, and dairy foods such as milk and ice cream. Dairy products contain lactose, which can be hard for some people to digest. If dairy foods bother you, try lactose-free milk.*

- **Eat smart.** Avoid heartburn-triggering foods such as spicy dishes, greasy foods, chocolate, caffeine, carbonated drinks, acidic foods such as tomatoes and citrus fruits, and mint-flavored foods. Trigger foods are different for everyone, so get to know yours and avoid them.

- **Loosen up.** Avoid tight-fitting bras and clothes that are snug around your stomach and chest.

- **Sit up after eating.** Remaining upright allows gravity to help keep stomach contents out of your esophagus. Try to wait at least three hours after a meal to lie down or go to bed.

- **Prop up your bed.** Stuff pillows under one end of the mattress so your head is a few inches higher than your stomach as you sleep.

- **Check with your provider.** If you still have heartburn despite making these changes, talk with your provider about using medication. Over-the-counter antacids that contain aluminum, calcium, or magnesium are usually considered safe during pregnancy, although they should be taken only according to dosage guidelines. Do not take medications such as ranitidine (brand name Zantac), cimetidine (brand name Tagamet), or lansoprazole (brand name Prevacid) unless your provider tells you to.

HEMORRHOIDS: SOOTHE THE ITCH

Hemorrhoids are swollen blood vessels in your rectum and around your anus. When blood vessels in this area swell, they can become itchy and painful. Sometimes they can even start to bleed, especially when you are constipated and push to pass hard stool.

Here are some tips for coping with hemorrhoids:

- **Don't strain.** If you're constipated and your bowels aren't moving as you'd like, take steps to get rid of constipation, such as eating more fiber and drinking more water. Straining to produce a bowel movement can aggravate hemorrhoids.

- **Move around.** Standing or sitting still for long periods of time can cause hemorrhoids to form or to worsen. Stretch and go for a short walk (even if it's only over to the window and back) every 30 to 60 minutes.

- **Cool down.** Use ice packs to reduce swelling and relieve pain.

- *Call your provider if you see blood in your stool.* Bloody stool can be a sign of other problems besides hemorrhoids. Your provider will want to check to make sure the bleeding is caused by hemorrhoids, not by something more serious.

- *Ask your provider about over-the-counter remedies.* Creams, ointments, and witch hazel wipes sold as hemorrhoid remedies are typically considered safe for pregnant women, but follow the directions exactly. Many are recommended for no more than one week of use.

COPING WITH MORNING SICKNESS

Morning sickness, which can come on any time of day, occurs most commonly in early pregnancy. It usually goes away by the end of the first trimester (around 13 weeks) when your body gets used to all of the extra pregnancy hormones floating around in your blood, although it does occasionally linger into the second trimester and beyond.

Although morning sickness can make you feel pretty crummy, it won't hurt you or your baby as long as you're able to keep down some food and water. Nausea and vomiting may prevent you from gaining the recommended 2 to 4 pounds during the first trimester, but as long as you're not underweight to start with, that shouldn't be a problem.

To cope with morning sickness, try these tips:

- *Keep something in your stomach.* Eat six small meals and healthy snacks rather than three large meals a day. Allowing your stomach to become empty can bring on nausea and vomiting.

- *Stay upright.* Avoid lying down after you eat, which can allow food and stomach juices to creep into the back of your throat and nauseate you.

- *Keep track of your triggers.* Pay attention to what foods, smells, and situations make you feel nauseated, and avoid them. For example, the smell of meat cooking on a grill triggers waves of nausea in some women.

- *Eat plain foods.* Bland foods such as rice, applesauce, toast, and bananas are more likely to stay in your stomach than rich, heavy, spicy foods.

- *Eat crackers in bed.* If you wake up feeling sick to your stomach, nibble on some plain crackers, dry toast, or dry cereal before getting out of bed. Get up slowly, because movement can make nausea worse.

- **Watch your water.** It's important to avoid getting dehydrated, because it's not good for your baby. Signs of dehydration include dark-colored urine, going four to six hours without urinating, and extreme thirst.

- **Vary your liquids.** If drinking water bothers you, try sucking on ice chips or popsicles; drinking weak tea, ginger ale, or watered-down fruit juice; sipping broth; or taking small spoonfuls of liquid every few minutes rather than gulping down a large amount of water.

- **Consider taking vitamin B$_6$ or ginger supplements.** Some studies suggest that they can help reduce pregnancy-related nausea; but check with your provider before using them.

- **Call your provider.** In rare cases, very bad morning sickness can develop into a serious condition called hyperemesis gravidarum (HG). Be sure to call your provider if nausea and vomiting become severe, you begin to lose weight, you become dehydrated, you are not urinating, your heart pounds or races, or you vomit blood. In the event that you develop HG, you may need to stay in the hospital for a few days and receive IV fluids and special medication. You should also call your provider if your nausea and vomiting are accompanied by fever, chills, sore throat, coughing, and body aches— you may have the flu, not morning sickness.

Q: *How do I know if I have HG?*

A: *Women with hyperemesis gravidarum (HG) have some or all of the following symptoms:*

- *Vomiting several times every day*
- *Vomiting after eating or drinking*
- *Feeling nauseated most of the time*
- *Having no appetite*
- *Feeling your heart race or pound*
- *Feeling faint*
- *Not being able to keep water down*
- *Going four to six hours or more without urinating*
- *Having dark-colored urine or no urine*
- *Vomiting bile (a greenish yellow digestive fluid) or blood*
- *Losing more than two pounds*

BACKACHES AND PAIN RELIEF

Have you ever noticed a pregnant woman leaning way back as she stood or walked? That's a natural response to weight gain in the belly area: as your center of gravity changes, you're likely to shift backward to balance the weight out front. It makes sense from a physics point of view—but unfortunately, it changes a woman's posture and puts lots of pressure on the spine.

Back pain can also occur when abdominal muscles weaken, as often happens in pregnant women. And when pregnancy hormones cause loosening of joints in the pelvic area to make room for your growing baby, that loosening can trigger pain in your back. Back pain may be accompanied by a condition called sciatica, which results when your baby's weight presses on the sciatic nerve in your back. Sciatica causes shooting pain that starts in your lower back and runs down the side or back of one leg to the knee or foot.

Be sure to call your provider if your back pain is accompanied by pressure or contractions in your pelvic area, if it's sharp and constant, or if it's accompanied by fever, bloody urine, and/or urgency or burning while urinating. These can be symptoms of a serious problem, such as preterm labor or kidney infection.

You can prevent or reduce back pain by following these back-care basics:

- *Watch your posture.* Focus on good posture when standing and walking, keeping your body straight and tall, with your chin tucked in slightly, your pelvis tilted inward, and your weight balanced on your feet.

- *Lift properly.* Get close to the object you're lifting, bend at the knees, grasp the object and hold it close to your body, and lift with your leg muscles as you stand up.

- *Sit correctly.* Sit in chairs that support your lower back. If a chair lacks low-back support, tuck a pillow or folded towel behind you for support.

- *Support your back while sleeping.* Sleep on your side with a pillow tucked between your knees to keep your spine in line.

Q: *Why do I sometimes have body aches?*

A: *As your baby grows and puts pressure on your bones, organs, and nerves, body aches can occur in your back, belly, legs, and groin. This is pretty common. Depending on what's causing the pain, you may find relief by lying down, walking around, or applying heat or cold.*

- **Be active.** Walking, swimming, and prenatal yoga help stretch and strengthen your back muscles.

- **Keep moving.** Avoid standing or sitting in one position for too long. Take a break and go for a quick walk every 30 minutes or so.

- **Stick with flat shoes.** Pack away your high heels for a while and instead choose low-heeled shoes with good arch support.

- **Relieve your pain.** Use ice, heat, and massage to help relax your back and reduce pain.

HEADACHE FIXES

Even if you don't usually get headaches, you might start getting them while you're pregnant. There are a few different kinds—and while you can't always tell the difference, knowing which kind could provide clues about how to deal with it.

Early pregnancy headaches During the first trimester, headaches can be caused by pregnancy hormones and changes in blood volume and flow. Your head may also start to ache if you suddenly cut out caffeine.

Tension headaches In the third trimester, tension headaches are common. These tend to occur when you can't get enough sleep, you feel stressed, or the muscles in the back of your head and neck are strained by posture changes that come from carrying so much weight around your middle.

Sinus headaches Pregnancy can bring on congestion and a runny nose in some women. When congestion builds up, it can irritate the sinuses and cause a headache around the eyes and cheeks.

Migraines Throughout pregnancy, hormone changes can trigger migraine headaches. A migraine is a severe headache that causes throbbing pain, often on just one side of the head. It may be accompanied by nausea and vomiting, chills, fatigue, sweating, sensitivity to light, or loss of appetite. Sometimes a migraine is preceded by what's called an aura, which can include any number of temporary visual disturbances such as blurred vision, eye pain, seeing stars or lines, or a reduction of peripheral vision. You may get migraines even if you've never had them before—many women get their first migraine during pregnancy.

Here are some ways to help prevent and cope with headaches during pregnancy:

- **Track your triggers.** Pay attention to your headache triggers, and avoid them. Migraines in particular tend to be set off by something you eat, smell, hear, or do. Common headache triggers include stress, bright lights, allergens, perfumes or other odors, changes in sleep patterns, exercise, loud noises, cigarette smoke, hunger, and certain foods, including processed or fermented foods, chocolate, dairy, pickled or marinated foods, citrus fruits, foods that contain monosodium glutamate (MSG) or nitrates, aged cheeses, smoked fish, nuts, onions, and artificial sweeteners.

- **Stay away from stress.** As much as possible, avoid stressful situations that may cause headaches.

- **Wet a washcloth.** Apply compresses (warm or cold, depending on which feels better) on your face, head, or neck.

- **Lie down.** Rest or nap in a dark, quiet room.

- **Relax.** Relaxation tools such as meditation, deep breathing, massage, exercise, a warm or cold shower, or pregnancy yoga may help with tension headaches.

- **Grab a glass.** Drink enough water. Being dehydrated can aggravate a headache.

- **Call your provider.** Check in with your provider if a headache is sudden, very painful, or the result of an injury; if you think you might have a sinus infection; or if it is accompanied by fever, stiff neck, vision changes, slurred speech, fogginess, numbness, sudden weight gain, pain in the upper-right abdomen, or swelling of hands or face.

Q: *Is it safe to take over-the-counter pain relievers during pregnancy?*

A: *Generally, acetaminophen (brand name Tylenol) is safe for pregnant women without liver disease, kidney disease, or other medical conditions— but take no more than is recommended.*

Nonsteroidal anti-inflammatory drugs (NSAIDs) such as ibuprofen (brand names Advil and Motrin), naproxen (brand name Aleve), and aspirin can cause bleeding problems. Because bleeding can be particularly dangerous around delivery, these medications are not advised throughout pregnancy, especially after 28 weeks of pregnancy.

When to Call Your Provider

Call your provider right away if you sense that something is seriously wrong with you or your baby, or if you experience any of the following:

- An injury or a blow to your abdomen or pelvis
- A significant decrease in your baby's movement
- Exposure to someone with chickenpox, mumps, or rubella
- Fainting or dizziness
- Fever of 100.4°F or above
- Flulike symptoms such as body aches, chills, fever, cough, congestion, and fatigue
- Intense itching over large parts of your body
- Jaundice (a yellowish discoloring of the whites of the eyes)
- Painful or frequent urination or urine that is cloudy, bloody, or has an unpleasant odor
- Severe headache or sudden changes in vision
- Severe leg cramping
- Significant depression, anxiety, or other emotional disturbance
- Sudden swelling, especially in your feet, face, or hands
- Sudden weight gain
- Trouble breathing
- Unusual chest pain
- Unusual gastrointestinal symptoms such as severe constipation or diarrhea
- Unusual pain or pressure of any kind, especially in the pelvis, abdomen, or lower back
- Vaginal bleeding, spotting, or unusual discharge or leaking of fluid
- Vomiting that is so bad you can't keep down any water or food
- Any other symptoms you find alarming

If you're concerned about something and not sure whether it's a problem, it's always better to call your provider's office, especially if it's during the day. Once evening comes, symptoms often feel worse, but by then your provider's office is closed and you may end up making a stressful (and possibly unnecessary) trip to the emergency room. If you call your provider when your concern first arises, you'll get an appointment, some advice, or reassurance that everything is fine. That will save you hours of worry and stress.

CHANGES ON THE OUTSIDE

Pregnancy causes all kinds of normal changes to your skin and hair. Some are kind of nice—women with thin hair usually enjoy having a thicker, heavier mane. But some are kind of irritating—acne is for teenagers, not moms! Here's what to expect:

Stretch marks As your baby grows, your skin stretches, and stretch marks may appear. These marks, which are pink, red, or brown streaks, are caused by tiny tears in the tissue just below the skin. They can show up on your breasts and belly, as well as your thighs and buttocks. They occur most commonly in the second half of pregnancy. You can lower your chances of getting stretch marks by avoiding rapid or excessive weight gain. Although there are many kinds of lotions and creams sold to prevent stretch marks, there's no proof that they work. After your baby is born, your stretch marks will likely fade, although they probably won't disappear entirely.

A dark line You may develop a dark line on your skin between your belly button and your pubic hair. That line, known by its Latin name, *linea nigra* ("black line"), is simply an area of skin darkening caused by your pregnancy hormones.

Dark spots Patches of dark skin (called chloasma, or the mask of pregnancy) may appear on your cheeks, forehead, upper lip, and nose. They may get darker if you spend time in the sun. Dark spots fade after you give birth, but they may not go away completely.

Acne Pregnancy hormones can cause facial pimples, especially if you used to get them around the time of your period. To help keep acne to a minimum, wash your face with gentle soap, and spot-treat pimples with an over-the-counter pimple cream that contains benzoyl peroxide. Don't use any other kind of acne medication unless your provider tells you it is safe. Some prescription acne drugs (including isotretinoin with brand names such as Accutane, Amnesteem, Claravis, and Sotret and other retinoids) can cause serious birth defects and need to be strictly avoided.

Itchy skin Pregnancy hormones and stretching skin can both cause itchy skin on your belly. It's also normal to feel some itchiness on the soles of your feet and the palms of your hands. Keep your skin moist by avoiding harsh soaps and hot water and by rubbing in gentle moisturizers a few times a day. Talk with your provider if itching becomes severe or you get a rash.

Skin tags These are small, soft, flaplike growths on the neck, armpits, and breasts. Your provider can snip them off if they bother you, although there is no medical reason to have them removed.

Varicose veins The weight of your baby's body puts pressure on your blood vessels and can partially block the flow of blood to your lower body. This can cause varicose veins, a condition in which the veins in your legs become swollen, sore, and more visible.

Spider veins The extra blood in your body, along with high hormone levels, can cause tiny blood vessels to turn red and form spidery patterns on your skin. These usually fade after birth.

Extra hair It's normal for the hair on your head to seem thicker and fuller while you're pregnant. It's also normal to grow extra (sometimes darker) hair on your chin, upper lip, cheeks, arms, legs, breasts, belly, chest, and back. That's because pregnancy hormones tell your body not to shed hair. During the six months after birth, your hair—on your head and elsewhere—will return to preconception normal, though it may then feel like you're losing an alarming amount of hair. Until then, it's fine to tweeze, wax, or shave unwanted hair. But avoid using bleach or chemical hair removers, which can be absorbed by the skin and carried elsewhere in the body (including to your baby) by the blood. We don't know if these products are unsafe during pregnancy, so it's best to choose alternate hair removal methods.

Nail changes Your fingernails and toenails may grow faster during pregnancy, or they may soften, break, and split more often. Either way, they'll return to normal after birth.

Breast changes A wide range of breast changes are also normal during pregnancy. Your breasts start responding to hormonal changes very soon after you get pregnant and continue to do so throughout pregnancy. In fact, sore breasts are the first physical sign of pregnancy for some women.

Typical breast changes include tenderness, fullness, heaviness, tingling, swelling, itchiness, and sensitivity. Because of an increase in fat tissue and milk glands, your breasts can grow by as much as a cup size or more.

As breasts get larger, the skin sometimes stretches enough that stretch marks appear. Bluish-colored veins may look bigger and more visible. Your nipples and the dark area around them, called the areola, may get darker and pointier and may develop bumps and an oily sheen. Toward the end of pregnancy, your nipples may leak fluid called colostrum, a sticky, yellowish liquid.

While some women enjoy the larger cup size, others do not. If the changes in your breasts are getting on your nerves, try these tips:

- **Chill out.** Apply ice or cold compresses to relieve pain and tenderness. (If that doesn't work, give moist heat a try.)

- **Get fitted.** Wear a supportive, well-fitted maternity bra that doesn't irritate your nipples. Cotton bras are usually best because they allow air flow around your skin and nipples.

- **Sleep in comfort.** Wear a comfortable sleeping bra if breast tenderness bothers you at night.

- **Use pads.** If your nipples are leaking, use breast pads to absorb the dampness.

- **Skip the soap.** If nipples are dry and cracked, avoid washing them with soap or hot water—just rinse them with warm water, let them air-dry, and apply a nonirritating moisturizer.

- **Speak up.** Talk with your provider if pain or swelling is severe or if you discover any lumps.

Congestion Nasal congestion, a runny nose, and even nosebleeds are common during the second and third trimesters of pregnancy. Hormone changes and increased blood volume can make the membranes in your nose either dryer or moister than usual.

Loosen congestion with saline nose drops, a warm cloth applied over the sinuses, and a steamy shower. (Don't take decongestants unless your provider tells you to.) If your nose is dry, drink more water and consider using a humidifier to add moisture to the air. Stop nosebleeds by sitting up, squeezing your nose between your thumb and your forefinger for a few minutes, and applying an ice pack to your nose.

Call your provider if your nasal congestion or runny nose is accompanied by flulike symptoms (fever, chills, body aches, sore throat, sneezing).

You may also feel a little breathless occasionally. During pregnancy, hormonal changes speed up your breathing. Because your lung volume is smaller as the baby's body takes up more space, you breathe more rapidly to take in enough oxygen to meet your baby's needs as well as your own.

Don't worry—unless you have asthma or some other condition that truly restricts your breathing and needs medical treatment, your baby is getting enough oxygen. To breathe easier, sit or stand up straight so your lungs have more room to expand.

Call your provider if your breathlessness becomes more serious or comes on suddenly, or if your lips, fingers, or toes start to look bluish.

STABILIZE YOUR MOOD

Expect to go back and forth between happiness and sadness, worry and calm, irritation and acceptance, fear and confidence, feeling totally in control one minute and dropping off into uncertainty the next. These feelings are all a normal part of pregnancy, especially during the first and third trimesters.

Mood changes have lots of causes during pregnancy. Hormones can rev up your emotions, especially in the early months. Tiredness, hunger, physical discomfort, weight gain, and stress can quickly sour a good mood. Many pregnant women also worry about whether they're going to be good parents.

Stress affects your mood, too. Feeling stressed about money, your job, family problems, your health, and all of the other concerns of life can make you feel anxious and blue.

Here are some ways to prevent and cope with mood swings:

- **Get enough sleep.** If you're having trouble sleeping at night, try to find time for a nap during the day.

- **Eat smart.** Nutritious foods and a healthy balance of carbohydrates, protein, and fat can help you feel physically balanced. Avoid skipping meals, because hunger can very quickly turn you from a lamb to a bear. High-sugar snacks may also set you off.

- **Get rid of as much stress as possible.** Some stress-causing situations can't be avoided. For example, if your boss always gets on your nerves, quitting your job probably isn't a viable option. But some stresses *can* be avoided. If your rush-hour commute makes you grouchy, carpool with a coworker or play relaxing music in the car. If you're stressing out about getting your daily chores done, ask family members to help.

- *Use relaxation tools.* Techniques such as deep breathing, meditation, and prenatal yoga can help you relax and feel less anxious.

- *Be active.* When you exercise, your brain releases chemicals that make you feel good. Walking, swimming, and participating in prenatal exercise classes are especially helpful.

- *Reach out for social support.* Having someone to talk to about your worries—a friend, a family member, or women in a pregnancy support group or yoga class—helps reduce anxiety and makes you feel less alone.

- *Tone down perfectionist feelings.* Sometimes pregnant women get overwhelmed by the expectation that they have to do everything perfectly—be perfect "hosts" while their babies are developing in the uterus and perfect mothers once their babies are born. Expecting perfection leads to disappointment and sadness, because being perfect is humanly impossible. Think honestly about the expectations you've set for yourself as a pregnant woman and a parent. Talk about them with your partner or a close friend. If your expectations seem unrealistic, try to reframe them in a more flexible way. For example, instead of thinking, "If I gain too much weight while I'm pregnant, I will be a failure," reframe your thought to, "I will try to gain the right amount of weight, but if I don't, I'll work hard to lose the extra pounds after my baby is born."

- *Ask for help if you need it.* A certain amount of moodiness is okay, but too much may be a sign of a more serious problem, such as depression or anxiety. Call your provider if your moods are extreme, if a disturbing mood lasts for more than two weeks, if you experience panic attacks, if you feel very sad, or if you are thinking about hurting yourself or your children. Talk therapy and medications (including antidepressant and antianxiety drugs that are safe to take during pregnancy) can help you feel better.

- *Don't take herbal remedies.* Herbs such as Saint-John's-wort, which is sold as a natural way to relieve depression, should not be used by pregnant women. Researchers don't yet know if such herbs are safe during pregnancy.

> **Q:** *Is it okay that my hands and fingers sometimes feel numb?*
>
> **A:** *Usually. The extra fluid in your body can press on nerves and cause feelings of achiness and numbness in the hands, wrists, and fingers, especially if you work with your hands or spend a lot of time at a keyboard. For relief, use cold compresses and take frequent breaks during which you open and close your hands and stretch your fingers a few times. The numbness should go away after you give birth. Call your provider if numbness is accompanied by sudden swelling of the hands or face.*

FLUID RETENTION: LET IT FLOW

Many pregnant women experience minor swelling, also called edema. Swelling is most likely to happen in the last trimester and can be worse toward the end of the day and in warm weather.

Swelling commonly occurs in the legs, feet, and ankles. This is because your baby's weight can press on certain blood vessels and cause a buildup of fluid in your lower body. Sitting or standing for long periods of time can increase swelling. Your hands and face may also swell.

Here are some ways to prevent and relieve swelling:

- *Move around.* If you have to stand or sit in one position for a long time, take frequent breaks. Get up, walk around, and stretch—this will boost your blood circulation and allow built-up fluid in the lower body to disperse.

- *Exercise.* Activities such as walking and swimming improve circulation and reduce swelling.

- *Cool off.* Cold helps relieve swelling. Take cold showers, float in a cool pool, use cold compresses, or spend time in air-conditioned rooms.

- *Elevate.* Put your feet up on a footstool, or lie down on your side with your feet raised up slightly on a pillow.

- *Loosen up.* Avoid tight clothing and jewelry, especially around the wrists and ankles.

- *Get support.* If swollen legs are making you very uncomfortable, wearing support hose may help.

- ***Avoid salty foods.*** The sodium in salt and processed foods can contribute to swelling.

- ***Call your provider.*** Get on the phone right away if one leg swells more than the other, if swelling comes on suddenly—especially in the hands and face—or if swelling is accompanied by severe headache, vision changes, dizziness, or belly pain, all of which can be signs of preeclampsia.

Chapter Eight

Making the World Around You Safer

There's a lot of news these days about dangerous chemicals in the environment. If you're pregnant, this is especially scary: you may have the feeling that you and your baby are constantly and inevitably surrounded by polluted air, dirty water, and contaminated food.

It can leave you feeling helpless—after all, you can't stop factories from belching clouds of smoke into the air, or companies from discharging chemicals into the water. Nor can you hold your breath for nine months or strap on a gas mask to filter the air before it enters your lungs.

Still, there is a lot you *can* do to protect yourself and your baby from environmental threats. You can make a huge difference, in fact. There are many steps you can take—most of them fairly simple—that greatly limit your exposure to dangerous toxins.

Many of the most potentially harmful chemicals in the environment are ones that you can avoid simply by educating yourself and making smart choices. When it comes to making the environment around you safer for yourself and your growing baby, you really do have more control than you realize.

Start by learning about what in your environment is unsafe—we've got you covered on that in this chapter, which includes information on common toxins to which you may be exposed. Then make a commitment to yourself and your baby to make choices that will protect you both during pregnancy and beyond—no gas mask required.

WALK AWAY FROM SMOKE

Even if you don't smoke, you and your baby are exposed to toxins when others near you light up and you breathe in their secondhand smoke. Cigarette smoke is full of chemicals that can contribute to health problems and pregnancy complications.

When it comes to making the environment around you safer for yourself and your growing baby, you have more control than you realize.

If you smoke, quit. If others smoke, shield yourself and your baby from their secondhand smoke by making your home, your car, your work area, and the space around you no-smoking zones.

Tell the people you work and live with that you want clean air for you and your baby and you simply cannot tolerate cigarette smoke near you. If someone in your proximity begins to smoke, walk away.

LOOK OUT FOR LEAD

Lead is a metal found naturally in water and soil. It's had various industrial uses, and for many years it was an ingredient in gasoline and some kinds of paint. As the dangers of lead became clear, the United States began to restrict its use significantly in the 1970s. But it remains in water and soil. Also, it is still used in some industrial and craft products, and it exists around us in products made before restrictions were tightened.

If humans get too much lead in their bodies—either through breathing or through eating—it causes lead poisoning. In adults, lead poisoning can

Q: *Is there a way to have lead removed from the body?*

A: *Once someone is exposed to lead, it is stored in his or her bones. A process called chelation therapy can be used to pull lead from the body, but the chemicals used as part of this therapy can have serious side effects. Chelation is typically recommended only when lead poisoning is severe. It is considered unsafe for pregnant women.*

cause permanent damage to the neurological system, kidneys, blood, stomach, intestines, and other organs.

Lead is even more toxic to children and unborn babies. Lead passes through a pregnant woman's body and into her baby, where even small amounts can be dangerous. Exposure to lead early in pregnancy can cause miscarriage, stillbirth, preterm birth, low birthweight, slow fetal growth, damage to the central nervous system, and developmental delays in an infant after birth. Children who are exposed to lead after birth can experience behavioral and learning problems, slowed growth, hearing loss, stomach problems, constipation, anemia, and other health problems.

IN DEPTH

Lead Safety Resources

See page 254

Although lead use has decreased in the United States, lead is still used in some industries. Because lead can make colors vibrant and bright, it can also be found in some types of craft and jewelry-making products, stained glass–making supplies, lead-glazed ceramic pottery, and a few types of oil and craft paint. Although most ceramic dishware made in the United States does not contain lead, hand-crafted ceramics and dishes made outside the United States may be lead-glazed.

Even small amounts of lead can be harmful because it accumulates in both a mom's body and her baby's body. Here are some ways to protect yourself and your baby from lead:

- **Be lead-safe at home.** If your house was built before 1978, when regulations regarding lead in paint were changed, it may contain lead-based paint. If lead-based paint is sanded or scraped, lead dust can enter your body through your lungs. Even if you can't see it in the air, lead dust can be released when lead-based paint is disturbed. Flaking or peeling lead paint should be removed only by a certified lead paint removal expert. While it's being removed, you (and any children who live with you) should stay away from your home until the paint is completely gone and all its dust has been properly cleaned up. If lead-based paint is safely encased—for example, if it's been painted over with nonlead paint and is not peeling—it doesn't have to be removed.

How to Check Your Drinking Water for Lead and Other Toxins

Drinking water providers are required to make the chemical profiles of their water available to the public. They do so in documents known as Consumer Confidence Reports (CCRs). These reports list the contaminants in the water supply.

To get a CCR for your water, contact your local board of health or municipal water provider or your state's environmental protection office. You can also consult the EPA's Local Drinking Water Information site (www.water.epa .gov/drink/local) to see if your municipality's drinking water quality report is posted. (If your drinking water comes from a well, you can have it evaluated yourself by a certified water testing lab.)

Water contaminants can vary from house to house because of the age of pipes and other factors, so even if your municipality's water gets a clean bill of health, you might also want to have the water that flows from your tap tested for purity. Your state health department can refer you to certified water testing labs in your area. Depending on how many contaminants you test for, a water test can cost from 15 dollars to hundreds of dollars.

If drinking water contains lead (more than 15 parts per billion), the Environmental Protection Agency recommends that children and pregnant women drink bottled water or water that's been run through a certified lead-removing filtration system.

If you have children under one year old, consider also having the water tested for nitrates, chemicals that can cause anemia. When children have anemia, their blood cannot carry enough oxygen for the cells in the body to work and grow well. Local health departments and environmental agencies can tell you how to find an inspector.

It's important to note that lead, nitrates, and other chemicals can't be removed by boiling your water. Boiling kills germs but doesn't remove chemicals.

- ***Be lead-safe at work.*** Lead is still used in some workplaces. Check with your human resources director or union representative to find out if there's lead where you work, especially if you are employed in printing, mining, jewelry-making, ceramic-making, smelting, auto repair, waste incineration, or the manufacturing of batteries, metal products, or ammunition. If there is lead in your workplace, talk with your provider about whether you can continue to work there; and if so, how you can protect yourself. If other members of your household work with lead, ask them to shower and change into clean clothes and shoes before coming home. Do not touch or wash their clothes or let their clothes come in contact with anyone else's clothes in the laundry.

- ***Use lead-safe dishware.*** Avoid using lead-glazed ceramic pottery and cracked dishes, as well as pewter or brass containers or utensils, which may have lead solder. If you're not sure about a dish's safety, don't use it. Avoid lead-crystal glasses, because they may pass small amounts of lead into the liquid they hold.

- ***Be cautious with internationally made goods.*** Lead use is less restricted in many other countries, leading to the importation of lead-tainted toys, jewelry, cosmetics, and even food. For example, lead has been found in some toys imported from China and candy from Mexico. Lead has also been discovered in internationally manufactured spices and in the seams of food cans from outside the United States.

- ***Watch for lead in unlikely places.*** Other possible sources of lead in the home include vinyl mini-blinds imported from other countries, old painted toys and jewelry, cosmetics containing surma or kohl, and certain folk remedies for upset stomach, including those containing greta and azarcon.

- ***Read labels on art and craft supplies.*** Some art and craft supplies, including oil paints, ceramic glazes, and stained-glass materials, may contain lead. (Lead-free acrylic or watercolor paints are safe to use during pregnancy and breastfeeding, but be sure to use them in a well-ventilated area.)

- ***Be safe after a storm.*** After a hurricane or flood, lead-contaminated floodwaters may get into well water or municipal water. Check with your local health department before drinking water after flooding.

- ***Have your soil tested.*** The soil in your yard may have been contaminated by lead from peeled paint or other sources. Although you are probably safe from contaminated yard soil, it will be a concern when your baby starts playing outside. Home lead test kits are sold in stores, but the Environmental Protection Agency advises against using them because they are not reliable enough. A certified lead inspector can test your soil. Contact the National Lead Information Center at (800) 424-LEAD (5323) to get contact information for lead inspectors in your area.

- **Eat to protect against lead.** Make sure you get enough calcium, iron, and vitamin C throughout pregnancy. These nutrients may help slow down the absorption of lead in your body, should you be exposed to it, and they may help prevent previously stored lead from being released from your bones and passed along to your baby.

- **Notify your provider.** If you suspect you've been exposed to lead, talk with your provider. A blood test can determine how much lead is in your blood. Your provider may refer you to an occupational health specialist for follow-up. As part of your evaluation, the source of the lead exposure will need to be identified and eliminated so that your newborn does not face the same exposure.

Q: *Should I avoid using pencils because they contain lead?*

A: *The "lead" in pencils is actually graphite, which contains no lead; so it's fine to use pencils.*

Q: *I've heard that there's lead in lipstick. Is that true?*

A: *Testing by the Food and Drug Administration (FDA) has found that many lipsticks do contain traces of lead, including some produced by Revlon, CoverGirl, L'Oréal, The Body Shop, Burt's Bees, Maybelline, Clinique, Avon, Estée Lauder, and Dior. The source of the lead seems to be color additives in the lipsticks. The FDA does not consider these lead levels to be unsafe because the amount of lead found was within FDA limits. Some of the lipsticks may be reformulated in the future—for example, Burt's Bees is working with its suppliers to find lead-free color alternatives. The Campaign for Safe Cosmetics website (www.safecosmetics.org) has more information about this. During pregnancy, the safest choice is to avoid wearing lipstick that contains lead.*

> **Q:** *Is it safe for me to paint my baby's nursery while I'm pregnant?*
>
> **A:** *It should be fine. There's no evidence that painting with today's lead-free latex indoor paints is unsafe. But it makes sense to take precautions while you paint. Work in a well-ventilated area, wear protective clothing, and wash paint off your skin. Stay away from any products that contain solvents, however. Solvents are chemicals that dissolve other substances. They include certain kinds of paint thinners, degreasers, and stain and varnish removers, along with some types of inks, lacquers, paints, and photography chemicals. Solvent exposure may increase risk of birth defects.*

CLEAR THE AIR OF CARBON MONOXIDE

Carbon monoxide is an odorless, tasteless, and colorless gas that is produced when fuel or other substances are burned. It is also an ingredient in cigarette smoke.

Although there is some carbon monoxide in the air we breathe, larger amounts can be unsafe, especially for pregnant women. Breathing in too much carbon monoxide prevents oxygen from getting into a mom's lungs and being carried by her blood throughout her body to her organs and her baby.

Signs of carbon monoxide poisoning include shortness of breath, headache, dizziness, fatigue, fainting, vomiting, nausea, confusion, and sleepiness. Carbon monoxide can damage the lungs, brain, and other organs, and in extreme cases can cause death. Fetuses whose mothers are exposed to dangerous levels of carbon monoxide can die or suffer brain damage.

Carbon monoxide is released when gasoline, coal, propane, kerosene, wood, charcoal, heating oil, or natural gas is burned by cars, generators, furnaces, fireplaces, wood stoves, ovens, and gas heaters and other kinds of engines, motors, and appliances. When fuel burners are in poor working order, used improperly, or vented unsafely, they can release carbon monoxide at a poisonous level. For example, carbon monoxide can build up dangerously in a house if a car is left idling in a closed attached garage without adequate ventilation, or if a charcoal grill is used indoors.

It's fairly easy to protect yourself and your baby from carbon monoxide by installing carbon monoxide detectors in your home. According to the U.S. Consumer Product Safety Commission (CPSC), carbon monoxide detectors are as important as smoke detectors; it recommends having at least one in the area outside individual bedrooms and checking the batteries on a regular basis. Detectors go off when carbon monoxide levels are high but not yet dangerous, so they can protect people from harm. If a carbon monoxide detector alarm sounds, the people in the house should leave and call 911. Carbon monoxide is odorless, so even if there are high levels in a house, people don't notice anything.

You can also stay safe by making sure all fuel-burning engines, appliances, heating systems, and fireplaces operate properly. CPSC advises having your heating system, including chimneys and flues, inspected every year.

AVOID MERCURY

Mercury is a metal released into the environment as a by-product of some industrial processes and when fossil fuels such as coal are burned. It accumulates in lakes, rivers, and oceans. When fish and shellfish in these waterways take in trace amounts of mercury, it builds up in their bodies, and when humans eat this type of seafood, they also ingest the mercury.

Many fish contain only small amounts of mercury. But very large fish that live a long time, such as shark and tilefish, eat so many smaller fish over the course of their lives that high levels of mercury can accumulate in their bodies. This doesn't pose much of a problem to nonpregnant adults, but for unborn babies, infants, toddlers, and children, even small amounts of mercury can

Q: *Is it true that there's mercury in lightbulbs?*

A: *Yes, in some; but it's a danger only if the bulbs break. Compact fluorescent lightbulbs (CFLs) contain small amounts of mercury sealed within the bulbs' glass tubing. If a CFL breaks, it can release some of its mercury vapor into the air. If you break a CFL, immediately leave the room and take any babies or children with you. Ask a nonpregnant adult to go into the room, open a window, turn off your central forced-air heating/air-conditioning system if you have one (to prevent the mercury vapor from spreading), clean up the debris from the broken bulb, and throw it away in an outdoor trash can. Then stay out of the room for several hours, leaving a window open and the air/heat system off.*

Q: *Is there mercury in dental fillings?*

A: *One kind of filling used for dental cavities is a silver-colored substance called amalgam, which contains silver, mercury, tin, copper, and other metals. The American Dental Association and the U.S. Food and Drug Administration consider amalgam safe, although there hasn't been a lot of research on amalgam in pregnant women, and some European countries advise against the use of amalgam during pregnancy. There are other kinds of fillings that contain no mercury. If you'd rather not have amalgam fillings, ask your dentist to use one of those.*

Q: *Is it safe to have my hair dyed or chemically straightened while I'm pregnant?*

A: *Probably. There appears to be no evidence that hair dyes or solutions used for perming or straightening hair are unsafe for you or your baby. Even so, it makes sense to follow a few safety precautions if you have hair treatments. Wear gloves if you're doing a treatment yourself, work in a well-ventilated area so you'll breathe in fewer fumes, and follow the directions on the product's package. If possible, choose hair-dying techniques in which dye is brushed onto the hair, not onto the scalp.*

be dangerous. Mercury can damage a baby's nervous system and cause brain damage, learning disabilities, and hearing loss.

Eating fish or shellfish with unacceptably high levels of mercury is the primary source of mercury exposure in humans. Because seafood offers many nutritional benefits that are important to pregnant women and their babies, such as omega-3 fatty acids, the U.S. Food and Drug Administration and the Environmental Protection Agency provide very specific guidelines about the types and amounts of fish that are safest for pregnant women. These guidelines aim to balance the benefits of seafood with the risks of possible mercury contamination. For a reminder of fish-eating guidelines, see page 54.

Other sources of mercury include nondigital thermometers and other medical and scientific equipment, although its use in these types of items is being reduced because of health concerns.

In the workplace, mercury may be found in dental offices and in the electrical, chemical, and mining industries, among others. If you are exposed to mercury at work, talk with your provider about how best to protect yourself.

TEST YOUR HOME FOR RADON

Radon is a radioactive gas that has no color, odor, or taste. It can leak from the ground, where it's produced naturally, into closed areas where people spend a lot of time, such as homes, schools, and workplaces. Radon enters buildings through cracks and holes in foundations, or along with water pumped indoors from a ground well. Buildings of any type or age can have radon. According to the National Radon Safety Board, 1 in 15 homes has elevated radon levels.

We know that radon hurts people by damaging their lungs. In fact, after cigarette smoking, it is the second-leading cause of lung cancer deaths in the United States, and the leading cause of lung cancer among nonsmokers.

We know much less about how radon affects unborn babies. But it's probably not good, so pregnant women should avoid it.

There are several steps you can take to protect yourself and your baby from radon.

- Start by checking with your local health department to see if radon levels are particularly high in your area. Even if they're low, you may have radon in your house; if they *are* high, that's good to know even if your own house isn't affected.

- Test your home for the presence of radon with a low-cost testing kit (sold in home-supply and hardware stores). Before you buy a test kit, check the label to make sure it meets Environmental Protection Agency requirements. Alternatively, you can hire a contractor to perform the test.

- If repairs are needed, look for a contractor who is certified by the National Radon Safety Board of the National Environmental Health Association.

The Environmental Protection Agency sells radon test kits and offers advice and information about reducing radon in your home. Call the National Radon Hotline at (800) 767-7236 or go to www.sosradon.org.

PREVENT EXPOSURE TO PESTICIDES

Pesticides and herbicides are chemicals used to kill or prevent pests such as insects, weeds, and fungus from interfering with the growth of crops or the safety of animals and humans. These chemicals can enter the body when people

Q: *Is DEET Safe?*

A: *Recommendations from the U.S. Centers for Disease Control don't tell pregnant women to avoid DEET (diethyltoluamide), an ingredient often found in insect repellents. But it's reasonable to stay away from it if you possibly can, unless you're in a situation in which using it makes more sense than not using it. For example, if you're camping in an area that's crawling with ticks or buzzing with mosquitoes, applying insect repellent makes a lot of sense. In that situation, the risk of getting Lyme disease or West Nile virus, which can be harmful to you and your baby, outweighs any theoretical risk that might be posed by the insect repellent.*

When possible, wear long sleeves and pants and try using safer (but less effective), natural bug repellents.

breathe them in, get them on their skin, or eat foods that have been treated with them. There's also pesticide and herbicide residue in the environment.

Examples of pesticides include sprays that kill mosquitoes, cockroaches, and pests that destroy agricultural crops; the liquid applied to dogs and cats to prevent flea infestation; and the creams used to kill head lice.

We don't know for sure what effect pesticides have on an unborn baby. In some studies, high-level exposure appears to increase risk of miscarriage, premature birth, low birthweight, birth defects, and learning problems. Although pesticide use is regulated by the federal government, there is a lack of agreement over pesticides' safety.

Despite what the research or the government says, it makes sense to stay away from pesticides while you're pregnant. Many of these chemicals kill other living things, so it's reasonable to believe that they could cause harm to your unborn baby, whose developing body and brain are known to be highly susceptible to other toxins.

The most cautious approach is to avoid pesticides whenever possible. Sometimes, however, the risk of using pesticides must be balanced with the risk of not using them. For example, if your home has cockroaches, it may be better for you to use indoor pesticides than to expose your family to roaches. In such situations, weigh the pros and cons, read and consider the warning labels on the pesticide package, and talk to your provider to help you make a plan.

Going Organic

We don't know for sure whether organic food, which is grown or raised without synthetic fertilizers, weed killers, and pesticides, is safer than conventional food. But it does harbor less pesticide residue.

Some women prefer to eat organic meat and produce during pregnancy. Some choose all organic; others buy a mix of nonorganic and organic.

To reduce exposure to pesticides and other toxins in nonorganic produce, wash it well and remove peels. (Keep in mind, however, that peels of some fruits and vegetables contain nutrients and fiber, so removing them may change the nutritional value of the food.) In meats, fish, and poultry, cut away any visible skin and fat, where pesticide levels may be higher.

Another option is to follow the advice of the Environmental Working Group (EWG). A nonprofit environmental advocacy group, the EWG ranks the pesticide residue typically found on 53 fruits and vegetables. It has compiled a list of "the dirty dozen" fruits and vegetables with the most pesticide residue and "the clean 15" with the least pesticide residue. For more information, check out the EWG's shopper's guide, www.ewg.org/foodnews/.

Whether you choose conventional or organic, remember that fruits and vegetables are packed with nutrients that are crucial for your health and your baby's development. Don't let fear of pesticides stop you from eating fruits and vegetables.

__The EWG Dirty Dozen:__ Apples, celery, sweet bell peppers, peaches, strawberries, imported nectarines, grapes, spinach, lettuce, cucumbers, domestic blueberries, and potatoes.

__The EWG Clean 15:__ Onions, sweet corn, pineapples, avocados, cabbage, sweet peas, asparagus, mangoes, eggplant, kiwi, domestic cantaloupe, sweet potatoes, grapefruit, watermelon, and mushrooms.

Since there's a lot we don't know about the health effects of toxins, chemicals, and other environmental contaminants, it makes sense to avoid using them whenever possible. You won't be able to prevent every exposure, but in this way, you are doing the best you can to protect yourself and your baby.

If you decide it's best to use a pesticide, use it in the safest way possible. For example, use bait traps rather than sprays. If you have to spray, protect yourself by leaving the area, having someone else apply the chemicals (or hiring a certified exterminator), staying away from the area for the recommended amount of time, following the pesticide package's directions regarding ventilation, removing all food and dishes from the area prior to pesticide application, and asking someone to wash all food-preparation surfaces after application has taken place. Pay close attention to any warnings, cautions, and restrictions on the product's label.

If you work in agriculture, landscaping, a veterinary office, a chemical company, or any other situation in which you are exposed to pesticides or herbicides on the job, talk with your provider about whether it is safe to continue working while you're pregnant, and what precautions you should take to protect yourself from the specific risks at your workplace.

ASSESS THE RISK OF ARSENIC

Arsenic is an element used to make some kinds of building products, glass, and semiconductors for electronics. It is released into the environment as a by-product from manufacturing, mining, and agriculture. Exposure to arsenic can raise the risk of miscarriage and birth defects. It can also contribute to lower intelligence in children.

You should care about arsenic because there may be some in your yard. Arsenic was used for years as a preservative in pressure-treated lumber, the kind of wood used to make backyard decks, some types of playground equipment, and other structures. Its use in residential areas was banned as of 2003, but many pressure-treated structures remain.

If you have a pressure-treated wood play set or deck built before 2003, the EPA recommends applying a penetrating stain or sealant to these items once every year or two to reduce your chances of coming in contact with arsenic. You and your family should also avoid inhaling sawdust from pressure-treated wood or smoke from fires in which pressure-treated wood is burned.

People may be exposed to arsenic if they work or live near metal smelters, live in agricultural areas where arsenic fertilizers (now banned in the United States) were used on crops, live near hazardous waste sites or incinerators, or drink well water containing high levels of arsenic. Well water can become

Q: *Is it safe to pump my own gasoline while I'm pregnant?*

A: *Probably. There's no clear evidence that pumping gasoline is dangerous for pregnant women. However, gasoline does contain toxic chemicals, so it makes sense to avoid exposing yourself to it. Whenever possible, ask someone else to fill your tank, or pull up to the full-service pump. If you do the pumping, avoid inhaling the gas fumes and wash your hands afterward.*

contaminated with arsenic due to its proximity to either industrial arsenic or rock that is naturally high in arsenic—as it is in parts of New England and the Midwest.

If you live in an area that may have high arsenic levels, you can protect yourself by limiting your contact with soil and getting well water tested for arsenic. (Municipal water is tested for arsenic by water suppliers according to EPA regulations.)

BE AWARE OF PLASTICS

Plastics contain a variety of chemicals, including phthalates and bisphenol A (BPA). Phthalates, a family of compounds that make plastic soft and flexible, are used in toys, medical devices (such as tubing), shampoos, cosmetics, and food packaging. BPA makes plastics clear, strong, and hard. It is used in baby bottles, food containers (to line metal food and beverage cans), and water bottles.

Hazards in the Workplace

The workplace is the primary source of exposure to toxic materials such as chemicals, radiation, dangerous metals, bacteria, and viruses. Be sure to confer with your provider if you work in potentially hazardous industries such as manufacturing, electronics, home remodeling, photography, dentistry, laboratories, printing, dry cleaning, human or animal health care, energy production, mining, or waste management. To learn more about workplace safety, contact the National Institute for Occupational Safety and Health (NIOSH) at www.cdc.gov/niosh or (800) CDC-INFO (232-4636).

Q: *Is it true that new clothing is treated with chemicals?*

A: *Fresh-from-the-factory clothing, bedding, and other fabric products may contain a chemical finish to prevent mildew and wrinkling. As an extra precaution, it's good to wash new clothes—especially baby clothes—to remove these substances before wearing them. The safety of chemicals used to make children's clothes flame-resistant has been questioned. However, the Consumer Product Safety Commission does not require sleepwear for babies under nine months of age to be flame-resistant because such clothing is snug-fitting and does not readily catch fire or burn.*

Research suggests that exposure to these chemicals before birth may lead to birth defects. Concern has been raised about the possibility that phthalates may raise the risk of defects in boys' reproductive systems and that BPA may have a negative health effect on the brain, behavior, and prostate gland in unborn babies, infants, and young children.

In 2009, the United States banned the use of some phthalates from toys and child-care articles, including any product that children age three and younger would use for sleeping, feeding, sucking, or teething. Some manufacturers have discontinued use of BPA in baby bottles. BPA exposure may also be linked to low birthweight and small size at birth. Prenatal BPA exposure has been linked to anxious and depressed behavior, hyperactivity, aggression, and poor emotional control in toddlers, especially among girls.

Studies are continuing on possible health effects of these chemicals. Until there are better answers, you can take these steps to limit your exposure:

- Stay away from BPA by choosing products made of BPA-free plastic, glass, polypropylene, or polyethylene. This means you shouldn't use plastic containers with the number 7 or the letters PC (for polycarbonate) in the recycling triangle on the bottom of the container.

- If you use BPA-containing plastic, discard it if it becomes scratched.

- Limit your use of canned food.

- Don't microwave food in plastic containers, pour hot liquids into plastic containers, or put plastics in the dishwasher.

- Once your baby is born, opt to breastfeed rather than use baby bottles; or use baby bottles made of glass, polypropylene, or polyethylene.

- Give your baby plastic toys only if they were made after February 2009 or are labeled phthalate-free.

- Limit use of baby lotions or powders that contain phthalates.

STEER CLEAR OF UNNECESSARY RADIATION

Unborn babies are vulnerable to the effects of radiation, especially during the first 18 weeks or so of pregnancy. Large amounts of radiation exposure increase the risk of birth defects and other problems.

However, medical X-rays tend not to pose much of a risk unless they are aimed directly at a pregnant woman's abdomen. Even then, the dosage in routine X-rays usually does not pose a major threat. X-rays of a woman's arms, legs, head, teeth (dental X-rays), or chest are generally safe during pregnancy because they don't expose her baby or her reproductive organs to radiation. X-rays of the lower torso—abdomen, stomach, pelvis, lower back, or kidneys—are more of a concern because they may put an unborn baby in the direct path of an X-ray beam.

To protect yourself and your baby, be sure to tell your provider that you're pregnant, and discuss whether the risk of having an X-ray outweighs the risk of not having one. Sometimes, routine X-rays (such as dental X-rays) can be postponed. If an X-ray is necessary, make sure the technician covers as much of your abdominal area as possible with a lead apron. (And don't worry about the lead in the apron; it poses no risk to you or your baby.) Dental X-rays use a very small amount of radiation, so the risk of them causing birth defects is very low.

Q: *Is it safe for me to have body scans at airports?*

A: *The imaging technology used by the Transportation Security Administration (TSA) in airports has been evaluated by the Food and Drug Administration and has been found to be safe for pregnant women. But if you would prefer not to receive electronic screening, you have the right to request alternative screening that includes a physical pat-down.*

AVOID AIR POLLUTION

Air pollution is caused by emissions from motor vehicles, factories, mines, power plants, and construction, along with dust and smoke. Pollution can be found in the air over bucolic rural areas as well as over busy urban metropolises, although it is likely to be denser in cities, especially on warm, sunny, still days.

Research suggests that some of the chemicals in air pollution, including carbon monoxide and polycyclic aromatic hydrocarbons (PAH), may increase the risk of premature birth. Air pollution may also contribute to reduced size at birth, along with anxiety, depression, and attention problems during childhood.

To protect yourself and your baby, avoid high-traffic areas while walking or exercising, stay away from airborne smoke and fumes, and keep track of local air quality so that you can stay indoors as much as possible when air quality is low. For updates on air-quality conditions and to sign up for e-mail or cell-phone smog alerts, check out the Environmental Protection Agency's AIRNow website (www.airnow.gov/).

Chapter Nine

Everything You Need to Know About Prenatal Testing

Your provider doesn't have a crystal ball, but there are a number of tests that can check on your baby's health while you're pregnant. These tests give many women the reassurance they need to worry less. And when there *is* a problem, these tests give moms and their partners valuable information that can help them and their babies.

Although most babies are born healthy, a small number (about 2 to 4 percent) are affected by some kind of a serious birth defect. A few of these birth defects can be treated or managed before, at, or after birth, improving outcomes for these babies.

It's tempting just to bury your head in the sand and put the thought of birth defects out of your mind. After all, the chances are very high that your baby will be just fine. Even so, it does make sense to learn a few things about birth defects and the tests that can detect them. Fairly early in your pregnancy, your provider will be offering you prenatal testing. Being informed about what those tests look for, how they are conducted, what their results may mean, and what choices you may face can help you make decisions that are right for you, your partner, and your baby. Even if you choose not to have prenatal testing, it's good to base that decision on solid medical information and the latest scientific research.

Knowing in advance about a birth defect gives you time to consider your reproductive options in consultation with your provider. You can also prepare yourself emotionally and arrange the best possible care during pregnancy and delivery.

MAKING INFORMED DECISIONS

Learning about testing can be empowering. Your provider can make recommendations and give advice, but decisions about testing belong to you. Being informed helps you make those important decisions.

Please note that the March of Dimes does not offer prenatal or diagnostic services or give directive advice or counseling. The March of Dimes provides information because of the belief that all prospective parents are entitled to the best information available to them about their own health and their baby's health.

Your provider can make recommendations and give advice, but decisions about testing belong to you. Being informed helps you make those important decisions.

Birth defects range in severity, even among affected babies. Some can be corrected with surgery or a blood transfusion. Others, such as neural tube defects, can be debilitating or even fatal. The known causes of birth defects include genetic problems (inherited from the baby's mother, father, or both), chromosomal abnormalities, and factors in the baby's immediate environment, such as a mother's medical conditions and infections during pregnancy and her exposure to tobacco, alcohol, drugs, and toxins before and during pregnancy. Many birth defects have no known cause.

A *combination* of genes and environmental exposure seems to cause some birth defects. In such cases, babies may inherit one or more genes that make them more likely to have a birth defect if they are exposed to certain environmental factors, such as alcohol, or if they lack certain preventive factors, such as the B vitamin folic acid (in the case of neural tube defects).

Some birth defects can be prevented, but not all. By getting good prenatal care and following the advice of your provider and the health recommendations in this book, you can go a long way toward giving your baby the best possible start in life.

TYPES OF TESTING

There are two main kinds of tests offered before and during pregnancy:

1. **Carrier screening,** ideally done before pregnancy, tests parents for genetic changes that could be passed to their future children.

2. **Prenatal testing** tests fetuses for birth defects and related health problems before they're born. This kind of testing can be broken down further:
   • *Screening tests* measure a baby's *risk* of having a birth defect.
   • *Diagnostic tests* determine whether a baby *actually has* a birth defect.

This chapter will cover both carrier screening and prenatal testing. (We'll tell you all about *newborn* screening in chapter 13.)

Let's start with a quick review of human genetics. Don't worry—we won't repeat your entire high school biology class! We'll just touch on the genetics facts you need to know in order to understand the tests you will be offered.

Your body is made up of billions and billions of cells. Each cell contains 23 pairs of chromosomes (46 in total). One set of 23 chromosomes came from your mother, and one came from your father.

Chromosomes vary in length, with chromosome 1 being the longest and chromosome 22 being the shortest. The 23rd pair of chromosomes represents the sex chromosomes; they determine the sex of a baby. A woman has two X chromosomes (as they're referred to in the alphabet soup–type notation used by scientists), and a man has an X chromosome and a Y chromosome. A baby receives one of the mother's sex chromosomes (always an X, because that's all women have) and one of the father's sex chromosomes (either an X or a Y). If the father passes along an X, you'll have a daughter; if he passes along a Y, you'll have a son. That's right—the father, not the mother, determines a baby's gender.

Every chromosome contains strands of hundreds or even thousands of genes. Overall, each cell in your body is home to about 20,000 genes. Genes carry information and instructions that guide your body's traits, development, and growth, as well as the functioning of every system in your body. For example, your genes determine your eye color and hair color, and they direct certain cells to become muscles, others to become blood, and so on.

Genes are passed down from parent to child on chromosomes. When you and your partner conceive a child, your egg (carrying one of each pair of your chromosomes) joins with his sperm (carrying one of each pair of his chromosomes), giving your baby 46 chromosomes—half from you, and half from your partner. Therefore, your baby has two copies of each gene, one on each chromosome.

One or both copies of a gene sometimes contains a change (also called a mutation) that can cause health conditions, genetic diseases, or gene-related birth defects. Whether one or both copies of the genes are changed and which copy gets passed from parent to child contribute to how birth defects are inherited.

Genetic-related birth defects can be difficult to understand. If you're confused, either as you read these pages or as you process the test results your provider gives you, take heart: genetics is difficult for most people to understand. That's why couples with genetic concerns usually meet with a genetic counselor or a doctor specializing in genetics. These providers have lots of experience explaining genetics to people without a science background, and they can help explain conditions as they relate to specific individuals. If your provider can't answer your questions, ask for a referral to a genetic counselor.

CARRIER SCREENING

Carriers of a genetic condition are people who carry (that is, have within their cells) one copy of a gene change that may cause a birth defect or medical condition in their children if a child inherits *two* changed copies.

Carriers have one changed copy of a gene and one copy of the gene that is typical, so carriers show no signs or symptoms of the birth defect or condition themselves. In these kinds of conditions, the inheritance pattern is called autosomal recessive, or simply recessive, meaning that two copies of the gene change are needed for the baby to be affected with the condition. In other words, the baby would have to inherit the gene change from *both* mother and father to be affected.

For example, a child can develop cystic fibrosis, a serious genetic condition that affects the lungs and digestive system, only if the child inherits mutations in the cystic fibrosis gene from *both* parents. If only *one* parent carries a cystic fibrosis gene change, a child will not develop the disorder. That makes cystic fibrosis a recessive disorder. Other examples of recessive disorders include sickle cell anemia and thalassemia (red blood cell disorders), Tay-Sachs disease (a fatal nervous system disorder), and several additional diseases that occur more frequently in certain ethnic groups, such as people of Ashkenazi Jewish (eastern European) descent. A genetic disorder occurs when a gene has a mutation, or change, that affects its action in the body. Simply having a gene is not associated with having a disorder. In fact, we all have many genes, and when they have no changes or mutations, they function normally.

Your provider can administer you and your partner a blood test to find out if either or both of you are carriers of gene changes that cause recessive disorders. This is called carrier screening.

Ideally it's best to have carrier screening done before you get pregnant. Knowing about your carrier status and your partner's carrier status helps you understand the risks that any baby you might conceive together would have of inheriting and developing a genetic condition. For example, if both parents are carriers of a gene change linked to a serious disorder, they might consider other conception options, such as adoption or using donor sperm or donor egg.

Here's how carrier screening works: Usually testing starts with the mom. She provides a blood sample that is sent to a lab to be tested. The lab analyzes the sample to check for genetic mutations for a variety of conditions known to be inherited in autosomal recessive fashion.

If the mom is identified as a carrier of a gene change for a condition, then the dad's blood needs to be tested to see if he is a carrier of a gene change for the same condition. Findings are sent to the mother's prenatal-care provider or genetic counselor, who discusses them with the parents and explains their possible impact on a future baby.

If carrier screening shows that both parents are carriers, there are three possible outcomes for a baby:

- The baby has a 1 in 4 chance of inheriting the gene change from *both* parents and developing the disorder.

- The baby has a 2 in 4 chance of inheriting the gene change from either parent alone, which means the baby would be a carrier but would not develop the disorder.

- The baby has a 1 in 4 chance of *not* inheriting the gene change from either parent, which means the baby would not be a carrier and would not develop the disease.

If carrier screening shows that neither partner carries gene changes for the recessive disorders that the test looks for, parents can feel reassured that their future baby won't develop those disorders. However, there is still a very small chance that a baby will be affected, as no test picks up 100 percent of mutations. In other words, carrier screening cannot absolutely guarantee that your baby will not have the birth defect in question.

If carrier screening shows that one parent is a carrier but the other is not, a baby they have together will have a 50 percent chance of also being a carrier. But such a baby will not be affected with the disorder.

A person's carrier status doesn't change over time, so you and your partner need carrier testing only once.

Some kinds of genetic conditions can be inherited when just *one* parent (who may have a mild or a more serious form of the disease) passes along a single gene change. This is called autosomal dominant inheritance. Each child of a parent who carries this kind of gene change has a 50 percent chance of inheriting the gene change and thus being affected with the condition.

Examples of autosomal dominant inheritance conditions include achondroplasia (a form of dwarfism) and Marfan syndrome (a connective tissue disorder). These kinds of gene changes are more common in pregnancies where the father is over age 40.

Q: *Carrier screening showed that my partner and I both carry genetic mutations associated with cystic fibrosis, which means a baby we would have together would have a 1 in 4 chance of inheriting the gene changes from both of us and developing cystic fibrosis. What can we do?*

A: *You have several options:*

- *You may choose not to get pregnant—perhaps to adopt.*
- *You may decide to get pregnant using donor egg or donor sperm from a donor who does not carry a cystic fibrosis mutation.*
- *You and your partner may choose to have pre-implantation genetic diagnosis. This means you would conceive via in vitro fertilization (IVF). Your eggs and your partner's sperm would be united in a laboratory dish; fertilized eggs would be tested for the presence of the cystic fibrosis mutations that you and your partner carry. If embryos result that do not carry those mutations, you may choose to have one implanted in your uterus.*
- *If you are already pregnant, you may request prenatal testing (either amniocentesis or chorionic villus sampling, which will be explained later in this chapter) to determine whether your baby has inherited the cystic fibrosis mutations from you and your partner; this will determine whether the baby will be affected. If your baby is affected, you can work with your obstetric and pediatric providers to consider your reproductive options and manage your pregnancy.*

Q: *Are there other genetic tests that may come up?*

A: *Yes, there are tests for genetic conditions that are generally rare and require evaluation by a geneticist.*

In another kind of gene inheritance, sons can inherit a genetic disease from a mother who carries a gene change on her X chromosome (usually with no effect on her own health because she has two copies of the X chromosome, unlike her son, who has only one). This is called X-linked inheritance because it is due to changes on the X chromosome. Because girls have two X chromosomes, they are less affected by a gene change on one of them than are boys, who have only one X chromosome. Each son of a mother who carries a gene change for an X-linked condition has a 1 in 2 chance of inheriting it. Daughters usually don't develop X-linked conditions, or they develop milder forms of the conditions, but they have a 1 in 2 chance of being carriers like their mothers.

Examples of X-linked disorders include hemophilia (a blood-clotting disorder), Duchenne muscular dystrophy (a progressive weakening of the muscles), and fragile X syndrome (the leading inherited cause of intellectual disability in the United States).

PRENATAL TESTING

Prenatal testing is medical testing done up to about 24 weeks of pregnancy to learn about the health of the baby. As noted earlier, there are two kinds of prenatal tests:

- *Screening tests,* such as blood tests and ultrasound, which are offered to nearly all pregnant women in the United States, tell a baby's *risk* of having a birth defect. Screening tests give parents-to-be an idea of the likelihood that their baby has certain kinds of problems, but they can't tell for sure. If a screening test shows that the risk of a birth defect is increased, parents can decide whether to have diagnostic testing. Because screening tests cast such a wide net, some findings will be false positive (the screening test is positive but the baby is actually unaffected), and some will be false negative (the screening test is negative but the baby is actually affected).

- *Diagnostic tests* are used to identify or rule out whether a baby actually *does* have certain birth defects. They can be done when screening tests indicate an increased risk, or simply because parents want to know for sure. Diagnostic tests include chorionic villus sampling and amniocentesis. These tests actually capture fetal cells for direct testing for specific conditions.

Screening Tests

Here's a look at the types of screening tests commonly available.

First-trimester screening A test called first-trimester screening combines the results of blood tests and the findings of an ultrasound. It is usually done between weeks 11 and 13. The American College of Obstetricians and Gynecologists (ACOG) recommends first-trimester screening because it can be useful in identifying pregnancies at increased risk for trisomy 21 (Down syndrome), trisomy 18 (Edwards syndrome), and trisomy 13 (Patau syndrome). It does not screen for neural tube defects.

Researchers have found that babies with chromosomal abnormalities such as Down syndrome can have increased fluid beneath the skin on the back of the neck. They have also found that the blood of women carrying babies with Down syndrome can have lower-than-usual levels of pregnancy-associated plasma protein A (PAPP-A) and higher-than-usual levels of a placental protein known as human chorionic gonadotropin (hCG). First-trimester screening takes all of this information into consideration.

Using ultrasound, your provider can measure the thickness of the fluid beneath the skin at the back of your baby's neck. This measurement is called the nuchal translucency and is sometimes abbreviated as NT. You will also be given a blood test for levels of PAPP-A and hCG. Using a computer program, your provider will combine the NT measurement from the ultrasound with the results of the blood test and your age. The program will then calculate the risk that the baby has trisomy 21, trisomy 18, or trisomy 13.

The result of a first-trimester screening is given as a fraction. For example, 1/1,000 would mean that your baby has a 1 in 1,000 chance of being born with one of the conditions that the test looks for. That means that of 1,000 women with this test result, 1 will have an affected baby.

First-trimester screening gives you an assessment of risk, but it cannot tell you for sure whether your baby is affected. The first-trimester screening test can detect Down syndrome in 82 to 87 percent of affected pregnancies. First-trimester screening can help you make an informed decision about whether to have diagnostic testing such as chorionic villus sampling (CVS) or amniocentesis, which we'll explain later in the chapter. An increased risk revealed on first-trimester screening suggests that parents consider CVS or amniocentesis in order to find out for sure.

To do an ultrasound in the first trimester, your provider (or an ultrasound technician) inserts a transducer that looks like a wand into your vagina;

the transducer sends out sound waves that create pictures of your baby on a computer screen. Because the fetus is very small at this point, inserting the transducer into the vagina allows the technician to get the closest and best possible images. The test has no known risks to you or your baby. The test can be a little uncomfortable, however, because in order to get the most accurate test results, your bladder should be full.

Multiple marker screening (also called maternal serum screening) During the second trimester, at 15 to 20 weeks, your provider will give you the option of having a blood test that looks at the levels of three or four substances in your blood which, if higher or lower than expected, can be signs of a birth defect such as Down syndrome, trisomy 18, or a neural tube defect. The result of multiple marker screening will tell you your baby's risk of having birth defects, but it can't tell you for sure if your baby actually has a problem. If the test shows an increased risk, your provider will suggest further diagnostic testing to learn more.

If the test checks for three substances, it's called a triple screen; if it checks for four substances, it's called a quad screen.

To do a multiple marker screen, your provider takes a blood sample from your arm. The sample goes to a laboratory, where levels of up to the following four substances can be measured:

1. **Alpha-fetoprotein** (AFP; a protein made in the baby's liver)

2. **Estriol** (a type of estrogen)

3. **Human chorionic gonadotropin** (a protein made by the placenta)

4. **Inhibin A** (a hormone)

Based on the levels of these substances in your blood, the test will calculate the risk that your baby has Down syndrome, trisomy 18, or a neural tube defect. If your risk is increased, you can opt to have an amniocentesis to find out for sure if your baby is affected.

Fully integrated screening A test called fully integrated screening, which combines first-trimester screening and quad screening, picks up 90 to 95 percent of cases of Down syndrome. The results of first-trimester screening and quad screening are analyzed by a computer program and made available to parents after the quad screen is done at 15 to 20 weeks. This provides the most sensitive testing—in other words, it picks up the most cases. However, you have to wait until after the quad screen to get your results. For women who don't mind waiting, this is a good option because it's the most sensitive screening test. For women who want earlier results, it's not as good an option.

Diagnostic Tests

Diagnostic tests are performed on genetic material from the baby to determine whether the baby has a genetic birth defect. Some women choose to have diagnostic tests following a screening test that shows increased risk, or even (because of factors such as their age) if a screening test shows average risk. Others skip screening tests and go right to diagnostic testing. In order to perform prenatal diagnostic tests, a provider obtains fetal cells in one of two ways:

Chorionic villus sampling (CVS) Chorionic villus sampling is usually done at 10 to 13 weeks of pregnancy. This is the earliest time in pregnancy that diagnostic testing is currently available.

To perform CVS, a provider takes a small sample of cells from the placenta, which has the same genetic material as the baby.

There are two ways to reach the placenta. With a transabdominal CVS, a provider inserts a thin needle through the mother's belly and into the uterus to take a small sample of placental tissue. With a transcervical CVS, a provider inserts a thin tube through the mother's vagina and cervix to take a tiny sample of placental tissue. The choice of approach is based on where the placenta is located and which approach will provide safest access to the placenta. If the placenta is in the back of the uterus, then a transcervical approach is better because there is no way to get at it transabdominally. If the placenta is located in the front of the uterus, then a transabdominal approach is typically used.

The tissue sample, called a chorionic villus sample, is sent to a laboratory, where the chromosomes in the cells are checked by performing a test known as a karyotype. A karyotype notes the presence or absence of all 23 pairs of chromosomes. It can also determine if the cells contain too many, too few, or damaged chromosomes.

CVS results come back in about one or two weeks.

If the results show abnormal chromosomes, that finding indicates that the baby has a chromosomal disorder.

If both parents are carriers of an autosomal recessive genetic condition, such as sickle cell anemia or cystic fibrosis, the baby's cells can be checked to see if the baby is a carrier or is affected by the condition. Similarly, if a particular genetic condition runs in the family, the cells can be checked for it.

After the test, women may experience cramping that feels similar to menstrual cramping, and they may have some spotting. Providers advise them to take it easy for the rest of the day, refraining from exercise and intercourse, and to avoid douching or using tampons. Women who have this test should call their provider if they have heavy bleeding or a fever, or if they start to feel contractions.

CVS carries a less than 1 in 300 to 500 risk of miscarriage—the same approximate risk as amniocentesis. CVS performed earlier than 10 weeks is associated with greater risk of miscarriage and limb reduction defects, so current guidelines advise against doing it before 10 weeks.

> **Q:** *What's the difference between CVS and amniocentesis?*
>
> **A:** *One major difference is that CVS can be done earlier in your pregnancy than amniocentesis. Also, CVS can be done through the cervix or through the abdomen, and amniocentesis is performed only through the abdomen. Both capture cells from the fetus on which karyotype and genetic testing can be performed. Both have a comparable rate of miscarriage: less than 1 in 300 to 500.*

Amniocentesis Amniocentesis is a test that captures cells in amniotic fluid to allow testing that will diagnose certain birth defects and genetic conditions. It is usually done between 15 and 20 weeks of pregnancy.

Amniotic fluid is the liquid that fills the amniotic sac and surrounds your baby in your uterus. Some of your baby's skin cells slough off into your amniotic fluid. These cells contain your baby's chromosomes and genes, which can be tested.

To perform an amniocentesis, a provider uses ultrasound to locate the baby, the placenta, and pockets of amniotic fluid in the uterus. Using the ultrasound as a guide, the provider inserts a needle through the mother's belly and uterus into the amniotic sac. The provider then takes a small sample of amniotic fluid—roughly 1 ounce—and sends it to a laboratory for analysis. At the lab, the baby's cells are grown for up to two weeks and then checked for chromosome problems. In addition, the fluid can be checked for levels of the substances alpha-fetoprotein and acetylcholinestcrase, which are elevated when the fetus has a neural tube defect. If there is a family history of a particular genetic condition or if one or both parents are carriers of a particular genetic condition, the cells can be tested for that condition as well.

During an amniocentesis, women may feel slight pressure or cramping in the area where the fluid is removed. They may also have cramping, blood spotting, or leakage of amniotic fluid afterward. They should take it easy for the rest of the day and call their provider if they experience bleeding, leakage of fluid, or fever.

Having an amniocentesis can increase the chance of having a miscarriage. The risk is small, however: less than 1 in 300 to 500 (about the same as for CVS, as noted earlier).

If I Have a CVS or an Amniocentesis, What Tests Are Done on the Fetal Cells?

Karyotype During the first days and weeks after a man's sperm fertilizes a woman's egg, cells divide rapidly and start to form an embryo. As cells divide, chromosomes are copied countless times from one cell to another. As this copying takes place, errors can sometimes occur. A cell may have too many or too few chromosomes, or chromosomes may get broken or rearranged. These chromosomal abnormalities can cause conditions known as chromosomal disorders. A karyotype test checks to see if there are 23 complete pairs of chromosomes in the fetal cells. Some examples of chromosomal disorders include:

- **Trisomy 21 (Down syndrome).** Three copies of chromosome 21—an extra on top of the usual pair—can cause intellectual disability, cardiac defects, and other health and development problems.
- **Trisomy 18 (Edwards syndrome) and trisomy 13 (Patau syndrome).** An extra copy of chromosome 13 or 18 can cause multiple birth defects, some of which can lead to stillbirth or be fatal early in life.
- **Sex chromosome abnormalities.** Missing or extra copies of sex chromosomes X and Y can cause sexual development disorders, infertility, growth abnormalities, and behavioral and learning problems. Conditions include Turner syndrome (in which a girl is missing all or part of an X chromosome) and Klinefelter syndrome (in which a boy has an extra X chromosome).

Single gene disorders If both parents are found to be carriers of the same genetic condition, such as sickle cell anemia or cystic fibrosis, cells from the fetus obtained by CVS or amniocentesis can be tested to see if the fetus is affected or is a carrier of that condition. This targeted testing is not done routinely on all specimens; it is based on family history and the parents' carrier status. Parents usually meet with a genetic counselor or a geneticist before having this type of testing.

Array comparative genomic hybridization (array CGH) Array CGH tests a baby's cells for over 100 syndromes (including Williams syndrome, Prader-Willi syndrome, and velocardiofacial syndrome) that are caused by deletions or duplications of small pieces of DNA on chromosomes. These changes are too subtle to be detected by the karyotype test. Each of these conditions is rare, but there are some instances where families might want to know about them—for example, if there is a family history of a rare genetic condition or if there are findings on ultrasound and parents want to know more about the possibility of a genetic condition. Talk to your provider and a geneticist or genetic counselor to see if you might want to consider array CGH testing if you are having a CVS or an amniocentesis.

TESTING BY ULTRASOUND

As an embryo grows, the dividing cells form bones, limbs, organs, and other structures. When this structural development is completed, the baby is known as a fetus. Sometimes structures don't form correctly, causing structural birth defects in the parts of a baby's body listed below. These defects can often be detected by an ultrasound (also called a sonogram) at 18 to 20 weeks.

- *The neural tube.* When the neural tube does not close properly, it can cause problems with the baby's developing brain, skull, and spinal cord.

- *The heart.* When parts of the heart don't develop exactly as they should, a variety of structural defects can occur. They vary from minor problems that can be repaired with surgery to serious defects that threaten a baby's ability to survive.

- *Cleft lip and palate.* Clefts in the lip and palate can cause feeding, speech, and cosmetic problems. Surgery after birth is very effective at correcting these conditions, known as orofacial clefts.

An ultrasound uses sound waves to show images of your baby on a computer screen. Your provider uses the pictures to look at your baby's body and check on your baby's growth, heart rate, and position. Ultrasound pictures also allow your provider to check on the health of your placenta, uterus, and amniotic fluid.

The March of Dimes recommends that all women have an ultrasound early in pregnancy, shortly after they begin prenatal care. This is to help confirm your estimated due date—information that may come in handy later in pregnancy to avoid preterm delivery— and to check to see if you're pregnant with more than one baby.

In assessing the baby's due date, this type of ultrasound is most accurate early in pregnancy. It is performed by placing the transducer in the vagina to get as close as possible to the fetus and obtain the best possible images. Later in pregnancy, ultrasound is less accurate in assessing gestational age and determining due date.

Around weeks 18 to 20, your provider will likely suggest that you have what's called an anatomy ultrasound or anatomy scan. This test looks at the entire anatomy of the baby and can reveal visual evidence of neural tube defects and other anatomical defects in the brain, heart, and abdominal wall. At this point, the ultrasound is performed by placing the transducer on your belly. If your provider suspects any anatomy problems, further testing or a meeting with a genetic counselor may be recommended. For example, if there appears to be a problem with the baby's heart, your provider would likely suggest a fetal echocardiogram, a type of ultrasound that takes a more detailed look at the baby's heart.

THE EMOTIONAL SIDE OF TESTING

Prenatal tests are more than just medical procedures. Because they seek information about your health and that of your baby, such testing can be very stressful.

These tests usually reassure you that your baby will most likely *not* be born with the birth defects in question. But getting worrisome results can cause anxiety at a time when you would prefer to be celebrating your pregnancy.

Planning for Delivery of a High-Risk Baby—and Beyond

Knowing in advance that your baby will be born with a genetic condition or birth defect gives you time to prepare in some of the following ways:

- *Consider seeing a maternal-fetal medicine specialist, an obstetrician who is specially trained to care for high-risk pregnancies.*

- *Talk with your provider about delivery options. Sometimes it's best to give birth in a hospital with a level III nursery—a neonatal intensive care unit (NICU)—which has the staffing and equipment to provide complex care, surgery, and life support for infants with special needs. (For more about nursery levels and NICUs, see page 20.)*

- *Ask your provider about the best way to give birth: a c-section is safer than a vaginal birth for a baby with certain birth defects.*

- *Meet with pediatric providers who can offer you information about the specialized care your baby will need after delivery, such as that offered by a pediatric cardiologist or neurologist.*

- *Learn about the kinds of treatment available to your baby after delivery.*

- *Join an organization or group that can provide you with support and education about caring for your baby's specific needs.*

> **Q:** *Is there any way to test for genetic conditions without invasive tests such as amniocentesis and CVS?*
>
> **A:** *Some companies are developing blood tests that would diagnose certain birth defects by isolating and analyzing fetal cells that are present in a pregnant woman's blood. Research is under way to determine how these tests may become part of prenatal care.*

You'll be informed by your provider of all options, and you will need plenty of support as you navigate your way through unfamiliar terms and health concerns. In addition to your obstetrician and a genetic counselor and/or geneticist, you and your partner may want to reach out to a clergyperson or social worker with experience helping parents of high-risk babies.

Some of that support also can come from March of Dimes' website (march ofdimes.com in English and nacersano.org in Spanish) and local chapters, which can help you find as much information as you need about your baby's condition. These sources can also help you find support groups that might allow you to meet with families in situations similar to yours. You can share your story and read about the experiences of other parents at marchofdimes .com/shareyourstory.

Chapter Ten

If the Unexpected Happens

Most pregnancies go smoothly. In fact, many women get through their pregnancies with nothing worse than a bit of morning sickness, an occasional backache, and a couple of bouts of constipation.

However, complications do occur for a small number of women. They develop anemia, high blood pressure, diabetes, or other problems.

We don't know what causes many pregnancy complications, although we often know the risk factors that are associated with them. For example, we don't know why one woman develops gestational diabetes and her best friend doesn't. But we do know that being obese, having slightly high blood sugar levels before pregnancy, having a family history of diabetes, and belonging to certain ethnic groups increases your likelihood of getting gestational diabetes.

Even though there's no guaranteed way to prevent pregnancy complications, there are ways to lower risk. The best is to go to all of your prenatal-care appointments. It also helps to keep existing medical conditions under control, eat well, take your prenatal multivitamin every day, exercise, gain the recommended amount of weight, and stay away from tobacco smoke, alcohol, and drugs.

KNOW WHAT TO LOOK FOR

Although it might be tempting to just skip this chapter, cross your fingers, and hope for the best, it actually makes sense to read it. If you know the symptoms of various pregnancy complications, you can call your provider and get treatment quickly if they occur. Early treatment can often help stop complications from developing or from getting worse.

Early treatment can often help stop complications from developing.

This is especially true with preterm labor. Some medicines can help prevent preterm labor for women who have had it in previous pregnancies. Other medicines help speed up lung development in babies that will likely be born early. Knowing the signs of preterm labor and calling your provider if any of them happen may prevent health problems in your baby and could even save your baby's life.

This chapter looks at the most common pregnancy complications. For each problem, we explain the possible causes, risk factors, symptoms to watch for, tests a provider uses to diagnose the problem, treatment options, and ways that moms can prevent or reduce their risk of having the problem.

Many pregnancy complications cannot be prevented, so women shouldn't blame themselves if they develop one. But, as with so many other situations in pregnancy, the choices a woman makes can have a powerful impact on her health and her baby's health.

ANEMIA

Red blood cells carry oxygen from the lungs to all parts of the body. Anemia occurs when blood doesn't have enough red blood cells, or when red blood cells are too small. Having anemia can deprive a mom and her baby of oxygen.

Anemia, which is usually caused by a shortage of iron, is common during pregnancy because the body must produce about 50 percent more blood to meet the oxygen needs of a growing baby. (Anemia may also have other, less common causes, such as blood disease or genetic conditions that affect the hemoglobin, which carries oxygen.)

Risk factors Pregnancy anemia is more common in women who had low iron levels or very heavy periods before getting pregnant.

If it happens Anemia can raise the risk of premature birth, low birthweight, and developmental delays.

What to look for Fatigue, weakness, headache, dizziness, faintness, chills, pale skin, numbness in the hands or feet, and shortness of breath.

Testing and diagnosis A provider uses a simple blood test to check for anemia several times during pregnancy, and more often if a woman has symptoms.

Treatment Women with anemia are usually advised to take an iron supplement. They can also boost iron stores by eating iron-rich foods such as lean beef and dark-meat chicken and turkey, lentils, dried beans and peas, egg yolks, dried fruits (prunes, apricots, and raisins), oatmeal, nuts, peanut butter, whole-grain breads, and spinach. The amount of iron the body absorbs from foods can be boosted by cutting back on caffeine and eating vitamin C–rich foods such as citrus fruits and tomatoes.

IN DEPTH
Health Advice for Moms of Multiples
See page 255

How to protect yourself Eat right and take your prenatal multivitamin every day.

BLEEDING

Bleeding can happen for many reasons during pregnancy. Sometimes it's a symptom of a serious problem, and sometimes it's not. During early pregnancy, it's not unusual to have some light, occasional spotting, especially after sex. Later, at the start of labor, it's also normal to have a small amount of dark blood mixed with mucus (called a "bloody show") pass out of your cervix. Heavier bleeding or bright red bleeding anytime during pregnancy is more likely to be a cause for concern.

Pregnancy bleeding can be caused by complications such as infection, miscarriage, ectopic pregnancy, growths on the cervix, placenta problems including placenta previa (a condition in which the placenta covers the opening of the cervix), placental abruption (separation of the placenta from the wall of the uterus), vasa previa (a condition in which the blood vessels that should be *in* the umbilical cord grow outside of it, where they can tear), or the start of labor.

Call your provider right away if you begin to bleed or spot. Your provider may perform an ultrasound, a pelvic exam, blood tests, or other kinds of tests to find out what is causing the bleeding.

CERVICAL INSUFFICIENCY

Cervical insufficiency (also called incompetent cervix) is a condition that occurs when your cervix (the opening of the uterus) begins to open too early, before your baby is ready to be born and before the contractions of labor begin. (Ordinarily, the cervix thins out and opens at the end of pregnancy, when labor begins.)

Risk factors Researchers don't know for sure what causes cervical insufficiency, but some possibilities include injury to the cervix during a previous birth or surgery, and the use of certain drugs. Having a shorter-than-average cervix appears to increase risk.

If it happens Women with cervical insufficiency have a higher risk of miscarriage and early birth.

What to look for Cervical insufficiency has no symptoms that can be felt by a pregnant woman.

Testing and diagnosis Transvaginal ultrasound can be performed to measure the length of the cervix and identify cervical insufficiency.

Treatment Your provider will probably recommend bedrest or cerclage, a procedure in which the cervix is stitched to help keep it closed until it's time for your baby to be born. You will most likely be advised to avoid sexual intercourse.

How to protect yourself Be sure to tell your provider if you've had previous cervical surgery or if you had problems with cervical insufficiency during previous pregnancies.

GESTATIONAL DIABETES

Diabetes is a condition in which the body has trouble using blood sugar effectively. Gestational diabetes (GD) is diabetes that develops during pregnancy (or "gestation") in a woman who didn't have it before getting pregnant. Having GD raises some health risks for a mom and her baby, but if she works with her provider and her prenatal health-care team to manage her GD and keep her blood sugar levels from going too high, she greatly improves her chances of having a healthy baby.

Risk factors The risk of GD goes up if a woman has any of the following risk factors:

- Age over 30
- Overweight or obese
- Higher-than-recommended pregnancy weight gain
- Family history of diabetes
- Ancestry in groups with higher-than-average rates of GD (African American, Native American, Asian, Hispanic, or Pacific Islander)
- GD or a large baby (9½ pounds or over) in a previous pregnancy
- Stillbirth in a previous pregnancy
- Prediabetes (also called impaired glucose tolerance, which means there is extra sugar in your blood) before pregnancy

If it happens Having too much sugar in the blood can increase a woman's risk of pregnancy complications. It also raises a baby's risk of large birth size and defects of the heart, spinal cord, kidney, and brain, and it raises the risk of newborn complications such as injury during delivery, low blood sugar, jaundice, and breathing problems. Later in a child's life, it increases the risk of childhood obesity and type 2 diabetes.

What to look for Frequent urination and excessive thirst, hunger, and fatigue (or it can have no symptoms).

Testing and diagnosis Providers usually check pregnant women for GD between the 24th and 28th weeks of pregnancy, or earlier if their risk is high.

The screening test, which is called a glucose challenge test, measures a woman's blood sugar after she drinks a very sweet liquid.

Treatment Keeping blood sugar in control is very important when a woman has GD. She can do this by following a special eating and exercise plan. Her provider may refer her to a diabetes educator or nutritionist who can educate her about blood sugar control and teach her how to check her blood sugar several times a day using finger-sticks. Sometimes women with GD must take diabetes medicine or insulin injections. Providers may recommend extra ultrasounds throughout pregnancy to make sure the baby is growing well.

GD usually goes away after delivery, but it raises the risk of getting diabetes later in life or in other pregnancies. However, exercise, eating right, and maintaining a healthy weight after the baby is born can reduce the risk of getting diabetes again in the future.

How to protect yourself Gain the recommended amount of weight, eat right, and be as active as your provider suggests.

PREGNANCY-RELATED HIGH BLOOD PRESSURE (WITH POSSIBLE PREECLAMPSIA AND ECLAMPSIA)

Blood pressure is the force of the blood on blood vessel walls. When that pressure becomes too high, a person is said to have high blood pressure (hypertension). Blood pressure is measured using two numbers, one over the other—for example, 120/80. The first number is the pressure when the heart is actively pumping blood, and the second number is the pressure when the heart is at rest between heartbeats. High blood pressure that starts after the 20th week of pregnancy is called pregnancy-related high blood pressure.

Risk factors These factors raise the risk of pregnancy-related high blood pressure:

- First-time pregnancy
- High blood pressure before pregnancy
- High blood pressure during a previous pregnancy
- Overweight or obese

- Pregnancy with more than one baby
- Preexisting medical conditions such as diabetes, kidney disease, rheumatoid arthritis, scleroderma, lupus, and certain blood diseases
- Age over 35
- African American ancestry

If it happens When blood pressure is high during pregnancy, a baby may not get enough oxygen and nutrients from the mother's blood. Having high blood pressure can cause pregnancy complications such as stillbirth, premature birth, and placental abruption, a condition in which the placenta separates from the wall of the uterus. It also raises your baby's risk of growing slowly and being born too small.

Most women with high blood pressure have healthy pregnancies. But about a quarter develop a condition called preeclampsia (formerly called toxemia), in which blood pressure continues to rise and the kidneys have trouble working correctly. In rare cases, preeclampsia can turn into eclampsia, a life-threatening condition (marked by seizures) that can cause damage to the mother's kidneys, liver, brain, heart, and eyes and can result in clotting and bleeding complications.

What to look for Headaches, dizziness, blurred vision, quick weight gain, swelling of the hands and face, pain in the upper-right belly.

Q: *What is HELLP?*

A: *HELLP is a severe form of preeclampsia that results in abnormalities in the liver and blood and can lead to bleeding problems. (HELLP stands for Hemolysis, Elevated Liver enzymes, and a Low Platelet count.) Symptoms, which usually occur in the third trimester or the first 48 hours after delivery, include pain in the upper-right abdomen, nausea or vomiting, fatigue, and headache. If not treated right away, HELLP can cause liver damage, kidney failure, bleeding problems, stroke, and even death in the mother, as well as placental abruption and premature birth. HELLP is diagnosed via blood tests that assess the blood (and its clotting function) and the liver. Treatment usually includes medication that controls blood pressure and prevents seizures; delivery of the baby may also be necessary.*

Testing and diagnosis Your provider measures your blood pressure during each prenatal visit using a cuff placed around your upper arm. Your provider also checks your urine for high levels of protein, which can be present when high blood pressure affects the kidneys' ability to work properly.

Treatment Delivering the baby is the only way to cure preeclampsia or eclampsia. Sometimes medications to bring down blood pressure or prevent seizures are given short-term, while delivery is planned. If the baby is too small to be born, the provider may give the mom steroids to speed up lung maturity in the baby and watch the mom's health very closely, either by checking her into the hospital or putting her on bedrest at home. After pregnancy, blood pressure usually returns to the preconception level.

How to protect yourself Gain the recommended amount of weight, be as active as your provider suggests, and go to all your prenatal visits so your provider can check your blood pressure and notice any rise in it as soon as it occurs.

PRENATAL DEPRESSION

Most people think of pregnancy as an exciting, joyful, even magical time. Fortunately, it often is. But sometimes pregnancy is not all sunshine and happiness. Being pregnant can trigger feelings of sadness and anxiety, especially when your life is unsettled.

If you are feeling depressed or suicidal, contact your provider right away, go to the hospital, call 911, or call the National Suicide Prevention Lifeline at (800) 273-TALK (8255).

Everyone feels sad or worried once in a while, but if these feelings occur frequently, you may have prenatal depression. If you do, you're not alone—10 to 20 percent of women become depressed during pregnancy.

It's important to remember that depression is not a pregnant woman's fault, and it's nothing to be embarrassed about or ashamed of. It is a medical condition that should be taken seriously, and that can be successfully treated. If you think you may be depressed, tell your provider.

Risk factors Depression can strike any woman, regardless of her race, income, age, education, health, job, or culture. Sometimes depression has no known cause, but it does occur more commonly in women with pregnancy-related worries.

For example, risk of depression goes up if a pregnancy was unplanned or if a woman had a hard time getting pregnant, has no partner or an unsupportive partner, is having pregnancy complications or a high-risk pregnancy, is pregnant with more than one baby, is a teen mother, or is carrying a baby diagnosed with a birth defect or health problem.

Depression is also more likely to strike if there is depression in the family or if a woman has a personal history of depression, bipolar disorder, anxiety, substance abuse, severe premenstrual mood swings, or physical or sexual abuse.

Other risk factors include having few or no supportive family members or friends, having financial worries, and experiencing highly stressful life events during pregnancy (such as job loss, death of a loved one, or having a partner in active duty in the military).

IN DEPTH

Getting Help When You're Depressed

See page 257

If it happens Pregnancy depression can impact a woman's ability to take care of herself, make smart choices for herself and her baby, and keep her prenatal-care appointments. As a result, it can increase her risk of many pregnancy complications and health problems for her and her baby, such as premature birth, low birth weight, and preeclampsia. Having depression during pregnancy also raises her likelihood of being depressed after her baby is born—a condition called postpartum depression.

What to look for Frequent bouts of crying, feelings of hopelessness, sleep problems (sleeping too much or not enough), loss of interest in favorite activities, fatigue, changes in appetite (eating too much or too little), anxiety, irritability, lack of energy, guilt, mood swings, persistent sadness, difficulty concentrating, lack of interest in the baby or pregnancy, and thoughts of hurting oneself or others or committing suicide.

IN DEPTH

Getting Help for Domestic Violence and Abuse

See page 258

Testing and diagnosis A provider will ask questions about a mom's mood and may have her fill out a depression questionnaire that measures the intensity of her feelings. The provider may refer a woman to a psychiatrist, psychologist, social worker, or therapist for treatment.

Treatment Talk therapy with a counselor or support group can often help. Antidepressant medication may also be needed. A woman may feel concerned about using antidepressant medicines for fear of harming her baby. However, there are several antidepressants that are considered safe during pregnancy. It is often more harmful for the baby *not* to treat a mom's depression, because depression can interfere with bonding and parenting. Having a healthy mother contributes to having a healthy baby.

How to protect yourself Get good social support and make self-care a priority. Ask your partner, family, and friends for support and for help with everyday tasks and challenges.

It can be difficult to reach out for assistance, especially when a woman is used to being independent. But having someone to talk to and an extra set of hands around the house can make life easier during pregnancy and after the baby comes home from the hospital. Do your best to keep yourself feeling good physically—eat nutritious foods, exercise, get enough sleep, keep all your prenatal-care appointments, and reduce stress as much as possible.

PRETERM LABOR AND BIRTH

Preterm labor is early labor that leads to birth before the 37th week of pregnancy. A full-term pregnancy is 37 to 41 weeks, but elective delivery should not occur before 39 weeks unless medically necessary. When babies are born early—even a few weeks early—they face a range of potential health problems. The earlier they're born, the greater their risk of complications.

Approximately 12 percent of babies are born before week 37 in the United States—a preterm birth rate higher than that of many other countries. (Babies born preterm are referred to as premature babies, or preemies.)

Risk factors Any woman can have a preterm birth. However, such births occur more often in women with certain risk factors, such as:

- Certain kinds of infections such as kidney infections and pneumonia
- Previous preterm births
- Pregnancy with more than one baby
- Certain problems in the cervix or uterus

- Conditions such as diabetes, high blood pressure and preeclampsia, and blood clotting disorders

- Pregnancy via in vitro fertilization (IVF)

- Vaginal bleeding

- Underweight before pregnancy

- Overweight or obese before or during pregnancy

- African American ancestry

- Age under 17 or over 35

- Closely spaced pregnancies

- Exposure to the drug DES

- Lack of social support

- Long working hours with long periods of standing

- Low-income status

- Exposure to certain kinds of environmental toxins

- Domestic violence and sexual, physical, or emotional abuse

- Habits such as smoking, using street drugs, or drinking alcohol

- Little or no prenatal care

If it happens Premature babies have an increased risk of poor brain development; of problems breathing, feeding, and digesting; and of dying in the first few days of life. Later in life, they are more likely to have developmental delays and learning problems. The seriousness of these problems is usually determined by how premature the baby is.

What to look for Contractions that make the belly tighten up like a fist every 10 minutes or more often; change in the color of vaginal discharge or bleeding from the vagina; the feeling that the baby is pushing down (pelvic pressure); low, dull backache; cramps that feel like a menstrual period; and belly cramps with or without diarrhea. One or more of these symptoms may occur.

If you have any of these symptoms, call your provider or go to the hospital right away. If you call your provider, he or she may tell you to go to the office or the hospital, or advise you to stop what you're doing and rest for a while. If the symptoms get worse or don't go away, call your provider again or go to the hospital. If the symptoms stop but come back, call your

Q: *When is a pregnant woman put on bedrest?*

A: *Providers recommend bedrest in hopes of preventing pregnancy problems from happening or from getting worse. Research suggests that bedrest is often of little benefit. Still, it is a precaution that many providers believe in. Some of the reasons a provider may recommend it include:*

- *Signs of early labor*
- *High blood pressure or preeclampsia*
- *Problems with the placenta or cervix*
- *Bleeding*
- *Pregnancy with more than one baby*
- *Swelling*
- *Oligohydramnios (low amniotic fluid)*

Bedrest can be recommended for anywhere from a few days to several months. Its extent varies, depending on the situation. Bedrest may mean anything from spending a couple of hours a day resting to staying in bed 24/7 and getting up only to use the bathroom.

If your provider advises bedrest, be sure to ask what activities you can and can't do. If you're on bedrest, you'll need lots of support from your partner, family, and friends, especially if you have other children.

provider again or go to the hospital. It may turn out that you're not in labor, but getting things checked out is okay. When it comes to preterm labor, it's best to be extra cautious.

Testing and diagnosis A provider does a pelvic exam and possibly an ultrasound to determine whether a mom is truly in early labor. If there are signs of preterm labor, the provider may want to give a test for fetal fibronectin (fFN), a protein produced during pregnancy. This test, which is similar to a Pap smear, checks to see if there is any fFN in the vagina and cervix. If the test finds no fFN, the woman probably won't have her baby for at least another two weeks.

Treatment Medications can sometimes slow or stop labor, at least for a short time. Corticosteroid drugs given before birth can help the baby's lungs mature, which can reduce health problems in the baby after birth. The sooner these medications are given, the better their chances are of working.

How to protect yourself Get good prenatal care, follow the self-care recommendations in this book, and call your provider right away if you have any symptoms of preterm labor. If you had a previous preterm birth, talk with your provider about using a type of progesterone called 17P to prevent another preterm birth.

MISCARRIAGE

A miscarriage is a pregnancy loss that occurs before 20 weeks, although it most often happens in the first trimester of pregnancy (up to week 13). Up to 20 percent of known pregnancies end in miscarriage; researchers believe that the true number of miscarriages is probably twice as high, since many miscarriages occur before a woman even knows she is pregnant.

Risk factors Most miscarriages are believed to occur when a pregnancy is not developing normally. The most common reason for faulty development is genetic abnormalities: about half of early miscarriages have genetic changes. Other factors that can contribute to miscarriage include health conditions in the mother (infections, diabetes, thyroid disease, hormone problems, autoimmune disorders such as lupus, and problems with the uterus or cervix) and lifestyle choices (having too much caffeine, smoking, drinking alcohol, and using street drugs). Often miscarriages have no known cause.

What to look for Vaginal bleeding, cramping low in the belly, passing of tissue from the vagina.

Testing and diagnosis Ultrasounds, pelvic exams, and blood tests help your provider determine whether you are having a miscarriage.

Treatment If your uterus empties itself out on its own, you don't need any treatment. If bleeding doesn't stop or your provider suspects that pregnancy tissue remains in your uterus, treatment may include medication or tissue-removing procedures such as dilation and curettage (D&C) or suction curettage.

If you miscarry, talk with your provider about how long you should wait to get pregnant again. Your body may recover in a month or two, after you've had one normal menstrual period. And be sure to have a full preconception

Emotions After Loss

Having a miscarriage or a stillbirth can be a devastating loss. You may feel sad, angry, guilty, disappointed, depressed, anxious, or all of these; you may cry, lose your appetite, feel unfocused, have trouble sleeping, feel fatigued, or lose interest in activities you used to enjoy. Or you may feel empty and numb. These feelings and reactions are normal. Here are some things that might help you cope:

- *Be patient with yourself, and don't judge your feelings in a negative way. It's okay to feel sad or angry. Also, remember that pregnancy hormones can impact your emotions; as hormone levels return to normal, you may feel calmer.*

- *Understand that your partner may be reacting differently.*

- *Ignore well-meaning people who don't understand your grief or try to cheer you up with insensitive comments such as, "It's better to lose the pregnancy than have a baby with birth defects," or "Don't worry, you can just get pregnant again."*

- *Take care of yourself physically. Even if you don't feel like it, try to get enough rest, eat nutritious food, and exercise. If possible, take some time off from work to give your body time to recuperate.*

- *Talk to family and friends. It can feel good just to discuss your experience with people who care about you.*

- *Reach out to others who have been through what you have. If you don't know anyone who's had a similar experience, look for online support groups.*

- *If you need more support than you can get from family and friends, ask your provider about support groups or grief counseling.*

- *Plan some kind of a ceremony or ritual so that you, your partner, and your family can say good-bye to your baby.*

- *If you are feeling depressed or suicidal, contact your provider right away, go to the hospital, call 911, or call the National Suicide Prevention Lifeline at (800) 273-TALK (8255).*

- *Give yourself time to heal emotionally before getting pregnant again. See your provider for a complete preconception checkup before you start trying to get pregnant again.*

checkup before you begin your next pregnancy. Most women who have a miscarriage go on to have healthy pregnancies.

How to protect yourself Most miscarriages cannot be prevented, and many happen due to genetic changes early in development that likewise cannot be predicted or prevented. So don't blame yourself. In general, though, you can lower your risk by being in the best possible health before getting pregnant and by making healthy choices during pregnancy.

STILLBIRTH

Stillbirth is a fetal death that occurs after 20 weeks of pregnancy, usually before labor begins.

Risk factors The following factors raise the risk of stillbirth:

- Problems with the baby (birth defects and genetic conditions such as Down syndrome)

- Placental problems (such as placental abruption)

- Umbilical cord disorders

- Cigarette smoking and cocaine use

- Maternal infections and chronic health conditions (such as poorly controlled diabetes, kidney disease, blood clotting disorders, and pregnancy-related high blood pressure)

- Untreated Rh disease

- Major trauma (such as from a car accident or domestic violence)

- Age over 35

- Overweight or obese

- African American ancestry

- Pregnancy with more than one baby

IN DEPTH
Less Common Pregnancy Complications
See page 260

What to look for Bleeding, pain, the absence of movement and kicking by the baby.

Testing and diagnosis An ultrasound can determine if a stillbirth has occurred, by revealing whether there is a heartbeat.

Treatment A stillborn baby must be delivered just as a live baby would be. The mother can choose to have labor induced with medications or to wait for labor to start naturally.

After a stillbirth, the provider orders an autopsy and/or certain tests on the baby, placenta, and umbilical cord to try to figure out why it happened. This information may help prevent problems in future pregnancies, although sometimes no cause is found. Many women who have a stillbirth go on to have healthy pregnancies in the future; however, knowing what may have caused the stillbirth allows a woman and her provider to take steps to reduce risk next time.

How to protect yourself Get good health care before and during pregnancy, keep chronic health conditions such as high blood pressure and diabetes under control, avoid and treat infections, and don't use tobacco, alcohol, or street drugs before or during pregnancy.

Chapter Eleven

The Checklist

Your baby will arrive before you know it. Are you ready? Use this checklist to make sure you and your baby get the very best start.

_____ Stock up on supplies.

You could spend several paychecks on supplies for your newborn—but all you really need are these important necessities:

- Diapers (up to 12 a day)
- Wipes (disposable or cloth)
- Diaper rash ointment
- A baby thermometer
- Petroleum jelly
- Cotton swabs or cotton to clean the umbilical stump
- A bulb syringe to suction mucus out of your baby's nose
- A nail clipper intended for infants
- Baby bath soap
- Saline nose drops
- Formula and bottles if you plan to feed your baby formula
- A breast pump if you plan to express breast milk

_____ Take childbirth classes.

Childbirth classes help you and your partner learn about and prepare for labor and birth. There are several kinds to choose from. Two of the most popular are Lamaze and Bradley, named after their developers. Most childbirth education classes use one of these two approaches. Many borrow elements from each.

Both the Lamaze method and the Bradley method teach women how to cope with labor pain. Both approaches encourage the woman's partner to participate in the labor and delivery process.

The Lamaze method teaches simple coping strategies for labor, including focused breathing, comfortable movement and positioning, massage, relaxation techniques, and labor support. Women receive information about medical procedures and pain relief during labor so they can make informed choices. For more information, visit the Lamaze website (www.lamaze.org) or call (800) 368-4404.

The Bradley method teaches natural childbirth to women with no medical complications. It emphasizes exercise, nutrition, and deep breathing. For more information, visit the Bradley website (www.bradleybirth.com) or call (800) 4-A-BIRTH (422-4784).

Other childbirth education techniques include the Alexander technique, HypnoBirthing, Birthing from Within, and BirthWorks. Learn as much as you can about each technique until you find an approach that seems right for you.

Here are some questions to ask before choosing a class:

- What method of childbirth education is taught?
- Is the instructor certified and up to date?
- What topics are covered?
- Are relaxation and breathing techniques taught?
- What is the instructor's philosophy toward pregnancy and birth?
- How big is the class? (Smaller classes with fewer than 10 couples are ideal.)
- Will the environment be welcoming and comfortable regardless of whether your childbirth partner is your spouse, your partner, a relative, or a friend?
- What is the class style: lecture or participatory?
- Are the time, length, and location of the class convenient?
- How much does the class cost?

To find childbirth classes near you, ask your provider and check with your health insurance carrier, your hospital or birthing center, and friends who have recently given birth. Another great source is the International Childbirth Education Association: www.icea.org or (800) 624-4934.

____ Learn about infant care.

Babies don't come with instruction manuals—but fortunately, many hospitals and pediatric offices offer classes that teach new parents the basics of baby care. Ask your provider or call your hospital to find classes near you.

To learn more, check out baby-care books in bookstores and libraries or look online at baby-care websites such as the March of Dimes site (marchofdimes .com or nacersano.org) and the American Academy of Pediatrics Healthy Children site (www.healthychildren.org). Stick with reputable books and websites created by trustworthy sources.

After your baby is born, the nurses will help you out and show you some hands-on baby-care basics. In addition, many hospitals offer a class in newborn care. And don't forget about family and friends, who will be happy to share their knowledge with you.

____ Educate yourself about breastfeeding.

Breastfeeding goes more smoothly if you've learned about it before your baby is born. Consider taking a breastfeeding class offered by your hospital or provider's office.

____ Decide on a pediatric provider.

Several months before your due date, start looking for a pediatric provider for your baby. Gather information about providers from family, friends, and neighbors. Your health insurer can give you a list of covered providers.

Remember that newborn babies see their providers frequently even when they're healthy, so you're best off going with a provider who has a location and hours that are convenient for you. During the first year of a baby's life, most providers schedule well-baby visits at two weeks, one month, two months, four months, six months, nine months, and one year of age. Providers check on a baby's growth, development, feeding, weight gain, and physical/cognitive milestones. They also give vaccines and educate parents about their baby's health.

Once you identify a provider who seems like a good fit, call and schedule a meet-and-greet appointment before the baby is born. During the visit, ask about the provider's education and training, office locations and hours, emergency coverage on nights/weekends, breastfeeding support, and any other issues you may have questions about. If you don't feel comfortable with the provider or the office, consider other options on your list.

_____ Line up a doula if you want extra support during labor and delivery.

Doulas are trained labor coaches hired by pregnant women to give emotional and physical support during labor and birth. They do not provide prenatal care, but they can be an additional support member on a childbirth team. Doulas specialize in giving advice on relaxation strategies, focused breathing, and using different positions during labor.

_____ Get your home ready for a new baby.

Before you bring your baby home, make sure your house is as safe as possible:

- Post emergency phone numbers—including those of your baby's provider, your local police and fire departments, and the American Association of Poison Control Centers' Poison Help Hotline (800) 222-1222—near every phone in your house, and enter them in your cell phone.
- Repair anything that could cause you to trip and fall as you walk around carrying your baby—for example, slippery area rugs, broken stairs, or loose handrails.
- Make sure your house or apartment number can be seen easily by firefighters, paramedics, or police.

_____ Prepare your family.

When a new baby joins the family, siblings—especially toddlers—may feel jealous or even hostile. You can help soften the blow by talking with your children about the new baby while you're pregnant and reassuring them that you'll continue to love them as much as you do now. Spend extra time together playing, reading books, and cuddling. Allow your children to get ready for their new sibling by helping you to decorate the baby's room and going with you to the store to buy baby supplies.

No matter how well you prepare, the first days and weeks may be bumpy, so ask a trusted friend or family member to spend time with your other children occasionally while you care for yourself and your baby. Also, be sure your home is thoroughly babyproofed if you have toddlers or younger children. Even if they don't grab electrical cords or climb on tables now, they may do so after their sibling is born, in an attempt to get your attention. Or they may get into mischief while you're busy changing a diaper or settling your baby down to sleep.

_____ Decide whether to bank your baby's cord blood.

Cord blood is the blood that's left in the umbilical cord and placenta after your baby is born and the cord is cut. Cord blood contains stem cells, which are cells that can grow into different kinds of cells. These cells, if preserved until needed, can be used later to treat medical problems in the baby or other family member. In fact, more than 70 disorders can now be treated with stem cells. Collecting cord blood is a quick, painless procedure. If not banked, cord blood is discarded.

You may bank your baby's cord blood in either a private or a public cord blood bank. Cord blood in a *public* bank is available to anyone who needs it. Cord blood stored in a *private* bank is available only to you and your family.

Private cord blood banks charge several thousand dollars for initial and yearly fees. The hospital may also charge to collect the blood for a private bank. There is no fee for public banking.

If you're interested, you must make arrangements about six weeks before your baby's birth. For public banks, you'll need to give a full family health history.

The following organizations offer information about banking cord blood:

- The National Marrow Donor Program maintains a list of hospitals that collect cord blood for public banks: www.marrow.org or (800) 627-7692.
- The Parent's Guide to Cord Blood Foundation provides listings of public and private banks: www.parentsguidecordblood.org.

_____ Consider making a birth plan.

A birth plan is a description of how you would like your labor and birth to unfold. It tells your provider whom you want with you during labor, whether you want to use pain medications, how to handle special religious or cultural issues that may come up, and whether (if you have a boy) you want him to be circumcised. Work on the plan with your partner during the weeks before your due date, and give it to your provider and to the nurse when you arrive at the hospital. Let your family know about your plan, too. But remember, it's *just* a plan, and you may need to be flexible once labor begins.

_____ Find out about health insurance.

If you have health insurance, ask your insurer about adding your baby to your policy. If you don't have insurance, coverage is available for many uninsured babies through the Children's Health Insurance Program (CHIP).

CHIP provides free or low-cost health coverage for more than 7 million children and teens up to the age of 19. The program covers U.S. citizens and eligible immigrants. Although it is a nationwide program, each state has its own CHIP program, and you must apply to your state program. For information on applying, call (877) KIDS-NOW (543-7669) or go to www.insurekidsnow.gov.

You may also be eligible for Women, Infants, and Children (WIC), a federal program that provides health-care referrals, nutrition education, and financial assistance for food and other needs for women and children with a low income, including pregnant women, breastfeeding women, and children up to five years old. Each state has its own WIC program; for information on applying, call your local health department or go to www.fns.usda.gov/wic/ for a list of WIC state offices.

_____ Buy a car safety seat.

It's hard to overstate the value of a car seat for babies. If you get into a car crash, even at low speed, any baby who is not in a car seat can be ejected from the car or thrown at high force against the inside of the car. Using a car seat restrains a baby within the car, offering important protection: correctly used car seats lower car-crash deaths by 71 percent in infants younger than one year old.

Babies should always ride in a car seat, starting with their very first ride home from the hospital. Inexperienced parents can sometimes find car seats difficult to install, so save yourself frustration by buying your infant seat and getting it set in your car several weeks before your due date. If you plan to take a taxi or car service home from the hospital, take your car seat to the hospital at the time of birth and let the taxi or car service know they'll need to allow time to install it. Most hospitals won't discharge a newborn to parents without a car seat.

There are many kinds of car safety seats available for babies and children of various ages and sizes. Infants should ride in a rear-facing car seat until they are two years old or until they reach the highest weight or height allowed by the car seat's manufacturer. If you can afford it, buy a new car seat. That way, you know for sure that the seat has never been in a crash. (Undergoing a crash can cause unseen damage to a car seat, making it less safe.) If you do choose to use an older car seat, make sure it's not more than a couple of years old, it's never been in a crash, it hasn't been the subject of a recall for safety defects, and it has its original instruction manual. To find out if a seat has been recalled, contact the Consumer Product Safety Commission: www .saferproducts.gov or (800) 638-2772.

Look for an infant car seat with a five-point harness (two shoulder straps, two leg straps, and one crotch strap). There are three kinds of seats that are approved for infants:

- *Infant-only seats* are for babies up to 22 to 35 pounds, depending on the specific model. (If your baby is born preterm and weighs under 5 pounds, you may need to buy a special insert; some manufacturers sell these to make their seats safe for tiny babies.)
- *Convertible seats* can be used facing rear for infants and then converted to front-facing seats when a baby reaches a certain age or size.
- *Three-in-one seats* can be used facing rear for infants, facing forward for toddlers and preschoolers, and as booster seats for older children.

Some seats have unique advantages; for example, many infant-only seats can be lifted out of the car and used as part of a stroller set. But all three types are equally safe, so choose whichever seems best for your situation.

No matter which kind of car seat you choose, be sure to follow the instructions that come with it and install the seat exactly as directed. It should fit snugly in your car and shouldn't move more than one inch in any direction.

If you aren't sure how to install the car seat, or if you'd like to check to make sure you're using it correctly, you can get help. Many local and state police departments, fire departments, and hospitals have specially trained and certified staff members who can inspect your child's car seat and advise you on using it safely, usually for free. Use the National Highway Traffic Safety Administration child seat inspection station locator (www.nhtsa.gov; click on "Child Safety") to find an inspection site near you.

_____ Make sure you have a safe place for your baby to sleep.

New babies spend much of their time sleeping, so it's important to have a safe place for them to sleep. Babies can't push or pull themselves out of harm's way if they become trapped or if something interferes with their breathing, so it's up to parents and caregivers to ensure their safety.

Bassinets and cradles may seem like good baby beds, but you can't count on them being safe, because their manufacturers don't have to follow federal safety standards, as crib makers must. For that reason, the March of Dimes recommends that the safest place for a baby to sleep is a new, full-size crib that meets all government safety rules. The crib should not have drop sides that go up and down. Although drop sides make it easier for an adult to lift a baby out of a crib, they can make a crib less structurally sound. Because of safety concerns, federal regulations no longer allow the sale or resale of drop-side cribs.

The crib's mattress should be firm and should fit tightly into the crib, to prevent your baby from getting trapped in the space between the crib and the mattress. (If you can fit two fingers into that space, it's too big.) Don't use bumpers, blankets, pillows, or anything else that could potentially trap or smother your baby, and don't place (or allow) stuffed animals in the crib. There should be nothing in the crib but your baby and the mattress.

Never allow your baby to sleep in bed with you or anyone else (often called cosleeping) because of the danger of falling, being smothered, or being crushed by someone. Be sure all of your baby's caretakers know this.

Bedside sleepers that lean against or attach to an adult bed are also considered unsafe: they pose a strangulation risk and have no mandatory safety standards as cribs do. If you want your baby close to you while sleeping, keep the crib in your bedroom during your baby's first few months of life.

If you do decide to buy or borrow a used crib, check it thoroughly to make sure it's safe. A baby can be injured or even killed in a crib that has loose or missing parts. You can learn more about safety-checking a used crib and find out if the crib you're considering has had any manufacturer recalls by contacting the Consumer Product Safety Commission (CPSC). Call (800) 638-2772 or go to www.saferproducts.gov and look under the "Search recalls and reports" tab. Millions of cribs are recalled each year for safety reasons.

___ **Take care of pregnancy paperwork.**

- *Triple-check your health insurance.* Investigate benefits, copays, deductibles, out-of-network vs. in-network coverage, and what kinds of referrals, restrictions, and approvals you'll need for prenatal care, testing, birth, and baby care.
- *Find out about maternity leave.* Your employer's human resources department should be able to provide details about your maternity benefits.

- *Sign a health proxy.* Check with a lawyer about signing paperwork that gives your partner or family member the right to make health decisions for you if you become unable to.
- *Get life insurance.* Buy insurance to benefit your baby in the event of your death. If you already have life insurance, check your coverage and buy more if needed.
- *Make a will.* Work with a lawyer or an online will-writing program to prepare a will. Close to the time of delivery, you can name a guardian who will have custody of your child in case anything happens to you and your partner.

Chapter Twelve

Go-Time

After months of waiting, preparing, learning, and dreaming, it's finally time for your baby to enter the world!

Childbirth is exciting, but it can also be scary, especially if this is your first baby. You may wonder how you will know when you're in labor and whether you'll be able to cope with the pain of childbirth. And if it's your second or third child, you're probably wondering how you will take care of everyone's needs after your new baby comes home, and how your children will react to having a new brother or sister.

Even if your pregnancy has been uneventful so far, you may be concerned about complications that could arise during delivery. You can't wait to meet your baby, but you may feel uncertain about how to care for a newborn and what kind of mother you'll be. These feelings are all completely normal— almost every pregnant woman feels them to some degree. Expect to have a roller coaster of emotions during your last few weeks of pregnancy.

With labor and delivery on the horizon, there are still lots of things you can do to keep yourself and your baby as healthy as possible. Continue to eat right, exercise as much as your provider advises, and keep all of your prenatal appointments. Practice the relaxation techniques you learned in your childbirth classes. Write down all of your questions as they occur to you, and discuss them with your provider. And finally, prepare yourself by learning about labor and delivery. This chapter covers everything you need to know on that front.

GETTING READY

You don't have to be a labor and delivery expert in order to have a baby; your provider and delivery room nurses will guide you through the process. Still, it's wise to have a well-informed understanding of what will go on once your labor contractions start, as well as possible complications that may arise.

Not knowing what to expect, or being surprised when something unforeseen happens, can cause unnecessary stress and tension. You want to be as calm and relaxed during labor and delivery as possible. Even if certain potential situations seem unlikely, it makes sense to know about them so you can work with your provider to make decisions about your care.

> *It's wise to have a well-informed understanding of what will go on once your labor contractions start.*

Many pregnancies end with vaginal deliveries; unless special circumstances indicate the need for a cesarean section (c-section), this is what you can expect. So if you're having a healthy, uncomplicated pregnancy, you might think there's no reason to read up on c-sections. But there is. The fact is, about one-third of women in the United States give birth by c-section. A lot of those women go into the delivery room planning to deliver vaginally. But situations can change quickly during labor and delivery, so even if you *intend* to give birth vaginally, it's good to learn the basics about c-sections. You certainly won't have time to read up on them while you're being wheeled into surgery!

The same is true of pain medication during labor. You may go into labor thinking you're going to deliver your baby naturally—that is, without any pain medication at all. That's fine if you can do it. But after your contractions start, you may change your mind—and if you do, it's better if you've learned a few things about your pain-relief options beforehand.

All this points to one more important thing to think about now, before you give birth. Try to be as flexible as possible during labor and delivery. It's great to have a Plan A—but it's good to have a Plan B as well. Keep sight of the most important goal: having a healthy baby and staying healthy yourself.

Congratulations—you're almost there!

KEEPING TRACK OF TIME

There are two ways a baby can be born: vaginally or by c-section. We'll talk about both here. We'll start with vaginal birth, then cover unplanned and planned c-sections.

Unless you have a planned c-section, your childbirth experience begins with contractions, repeated tightening of the muscles of the uterus. Your body uses contractions to move your baby down into the pelvis, and then to push your baby out through the birth canal.

You might have some irregular contractions that occur days, weeks, or even months before your baby is born—contractions that do not become strong and regular with time, but rather come and go. These are called Braxton Hicks contractions, or false labor. They don't cause cervical change or lead to delivery.

How can you recognize true labor contractions? In general, labor contractions progress in a steadily increasing pattern. At first they are short, less intense, and widely spaced, but as labor progresses, they become longer, more intense, and closer together. When you have a contraction, your belly feels hard; when the contraction stops, your belly feels soft.

Here's a summary of ways to recognize true labor contractions:

- **They get more uncomfortable over time.** When labor contractions start, you may be able to walk and talk through them, but as they progress and get stronger and closer together, you will usually have to stop everything you're doing and breathe or count through each contraction.

- **They may move.** Labor contractions often start in the back of your body and move around to the front.

- **They get longer.** Early labor contractions may last about 30 seconds; as labor progresses, contractions last up to 60 seconds.

- **They get closer together.** Labor contractions get steadily closer together over time and happen in a pattern. For example, they may come every 20 minutes early in labor, and then increase to every 3 minutes as time goes on.

When you have contractions, use a watch or clock to time them. Write down the time when each contraction begins and ends so you know how long they last and how frequently they occur. Time them from the beginning of one contraction to the beginning of the next.

When your contractions are about 10 minutes apart, call your provider, who will help you decide whether it's time to go to the hospital. Providers usually know by a woman's voice on the phone whether it's time for her to go to the hospital. If the woman can chat easily, it's probably not time, but if she has to stop talking because she's having a contraction, the provider will probably tell her to head to the hospital.

At some point in your labor, your water will break. This occurrence is also called rupture of membranes. When this happens, the amniotic sac (bag) opens, releasing amniotic fluid (the "water") surrounding your baby.

Your water can break at any of various times: several hours before contractions begin, sometime during labor, or shortly before your baby is born. (If it doesn't break on its own, your doctor may poke the amniotic sac open with a small hook.) When the sac is opened, amniotic fluid flows out in a gush or a trickle, depending on how your baby is positioned. If it's a gush, it may seem like a lot of fluid, but it's only a couple of ounces.

Healthy pregnancy lasts about 40 weeks (280 days) from the first day of your last menstrual period. If your pregnancy is healthy, you should wait for normal labor to begin on its own.

If your water breaks before you go to the hospital, pay attention to its color and odor. Normal fluid is a clear yellow, much like urine (in fact, it contains your baby's urine), and often has white flecks called vernix. However, it can also be green, dark yellow, or brown. If it's a darker color, tell your provider, because it may mean your baby has already passed his or her first bowel movement (called meconium). Your provider will know to suction it out of your baby's lungs before your baby takes a first breath. If the fluid has an unpleasant odor, your provider will probably want to test it to see if there is an infection.

> **Q:** *What is nesting, and does it really happen?*
>
> **A:** *Nesting is the desire—sometimes accompanied by a burst of energy—to clean, cook, decorate, and organize your home during the days and weeks before your baby is born. Not all women feel it. If you develop an urge to clean behind the sofa, cook a half dozen casseroles, or paint your bathroom, take care not to overexert yourself, fall, or strain your back.*

Sometimes it can be hard to tell if your water has broken or if you're just leaking urine, which commonly occurs near the end of pregnancy. If the trickle of fluid is ongoing and you're uncertain what it is, wear a pad to collect some of the fluid. Look at the pad after you've worn it for about an hour. If the discharge looks and smells like urine, which has a distinctive odor, your water probably hasn't broken yet. If the pad contains a little bit of dark blood mixed with mucus, don't be alarmed. What you see is probably the mucus plug, also called the bloody show, which is the discharge that comes out of the cervix as it starts to open. But the emergence of the mucus plug doesn't necessarily mean your water has broken.

Heavy vaginal bleeding is not normal during labor, so definitely call your provider and go directly to the hospital if you have heavy, bright-red vaginal bleeding. Also call your provider if your water breaks and you don't go into labor. You'll probably be advised to go to the hospital for monitoring, to start antibiotics, and to start medications to induce labor. Once your water breaks, the risk of infection increases, so it's important to make arrangements with your provider to get labor going safely.

INDUCING LABOR

If labor doesn't begin naturally, or if it starts and then stops, your provider may decide to kick-start it. This is called inducing labor.

Inducing labor does have some risks, including infection, uterine rupture, and an increased risk of c-section, so it should be done only when there are medical reasons for it. Some of those reasons include:

- The placenta develops problems.
- High blood pressure, preeclampsia, or eclampsia occur.
- The amniotic sac has broken, but contractions haven't begun.
- The baby is overdue (usually between 41 and 42 weeks) and there is concern about his or her well-being.

Typically, a provider will not induce labor unless a woman's cervix is "ripe"—meaning it is soft, thin (effaced), and open (dilated) enough for labor to begin. (Providers use a scoring system called the Bishop score to determine whether the cervix is ready for labor.) If induction is necessary and the cervix is not ripe enough, a provider can use certain drugs or a balloon-like medical device to help it ripen.

There are three ways to induce labor:

1. By giving an intravenous infusion of oxytocin (brand name Pitocin), a hormone drug that can start or speed up contractions. Oxytocin works quickly—usually within 30 minutes.

Q: *What does it mean that a baby is in the "breech" position?*

A: *Babies typically move into a head-down position during the last month or so of pregnancy. But some don't, meaning that when labor starts, they are positioned to be born feet-first or buttocks-first. This is called the breech position. Having a breech baby is most likely to happen when a woman goes into labor early, has had previous pregnancies, is pregnant with more than one baby, has a condition in which there is too little fluid in the amniotic sac, or has problems or abnormalities with the uterus or placenta. Sometimes it happens for no identifiable reason.*

If your baby is breech, your provider may recommend a procedure called an external cephalic version. In this procedure, a provider places his or her hands on your belly and tries to move the baby into a head-down position from the outside of your body. This can be uncomfortable, and it may not work. Sometimes a "version," as it is often called, is attempted more than once. Delivering a breech baby vaginally is risky, especially for mothers having their first delivery, so if your baby can't be moved out of the breech position, your provider will likely recommend a c-section.

---

2. By doing a procedure called "stripping the membranes." In this procedure, your provider sweeps a gloved finger along the membrane between the amniotic sac and the uterus. This can sometimes help your body start labor.

3. By rupturing the amniotic sac. Using a hooklike medical tool, your provider can make a hole in the amniotic sac. This procedure sometimes causes contractions to start or speed up.

COPING WITH PAIN

There's no way around it: you're going to feel pain while giving birth. But there's no telling how much pain you'll have. And almost all women feel that the pain is worth it once they hold their beautiful newborn for the first time.

During labor and delivery, there are two ways to relieve pain: with relaxation techniques and with pain medication. It's good to know about both options so you can use them as needed.

The amount of pain you feel depends on many factors, including your own ability to withstand pain, your health history, the length of your labor, the strength of your contractions, the size and position of your baby, and whether you are tired or well rested before labor begins.

Psychological factors also play a part in how you feel pain. Studies suggest that pain feels worse in women who are especially tense or fearful about giving birth, have little or no social support during pregnancy and delivery, or who feel unprepared for birth. On the flip side, women with lots of support who feel well prepared for birth and feel relaxed and confident report feeling less pain.

During labor and delivery, there are two ways to relieve pain: with relaxation techniques and with pain medication. It's good to know about both options so you can use them as needed.

Relaxation techniques The relaxation techniques often used by women in labor include breathing exercises, massage, visualization (focusing on a relaxing image, such as a sandy beach), music (listening to favorite quiet selections), guided meditation (listening to a recording of a trained mind/

Q: *What is back labor?*

A: *Babies are usually face-down (looking toward the mother's spine) as they move into the pelvis. But sometimes a baby is face-up (looking toward the mother's belly) instead. This can cause intense back pain during labor and is called back labor. If you're having back labor, your provider may try to rotate your baby by having you change positions, although that doesn't always work. Sometimes babies rotate (either in response to a mother's changed position or on their own), and sometimes unrotated babies are delivered face-up.*

body expert guiding you through a meditation session), hydrotherapy (warm showers or baths), and progressive relaxation (mindfully relaxing each of your muscle groups, starting with the top of your head and progressing to the tips of your toes). You can learn about relaxation techniques in childbirth classes, in books, on websites, and on DVDs.

Pain medications The different pain medications available offer varying amounts of relief. They are a safe way to make labor more comfortable.

Women tend to have strong opinions when it comes to labor pain relief. Having a preference about whether you do or don't want to use pain medication is fine, but it's wise not to be too rigid. Some women want to have a natural, medication-free childbirth, and if all goes well, that's terrific. But if they decide the pain is too much and medication would make the experience better, that's okay, too. At the same time, some women want their epidural early—if possible, they'd have it in the hospital parking lot! But if they arrive in the delivery room fully dilated, ready to push, and too late for pain medication, they are sometimes surprised at what they can handle. The bottom line is this: make a plan, but keep an open mind. You never know what labor is going to throw your way.

Women with lots of support who feel well prepared for birth and feel relaxed and confident report feeling less pain.

The following chart explains the pain medications available during labor and delivery, along with the pros and cons of each type. Choices may vary at your hospital, so ask your provider about the pain medications that will be available to you when you give birth.

Medication	Pros	Cons
Narcotic (opioid) medication Medication injected through an IV or into muscle	Takes the edge off pain but still allows you to push; can be taken early in labor while allowing for an epidural later, if needed	Helps for a short time only, can make you sleepy, and can have annoying side effects (nausea, vomiting, itchiness, shivering); if given too close to delivery, can lower baby's heart rate, breathing, and ability to latch on during early breastfeeding
Epidural anesthesia Medication given continuously through a tube that is inserted by needle into a space below your spinal cord in your lower back; the most popular and effective kind of pain relief used during labor—more than half of women who give birth in U.S. hospitals have an epidural	Numbs your lower body so you can't feel the pain from contractions; you remain awake but feel very little pain—dosage can be adjusted during labor as needed	Has delay in effectiveness (pain relief doesn't start for 10 to 20 minutes); can limit your ability to move or walk around during labor; causes very bad headache after delivery in about 1 percent of women
Spinal block Anesthesia medication injected into the spinal fluid in your lower back	Allows you to remain awake but feel very little pain; gives relief as soon as the medication is injected	Usually can be given only once during labor, and lasts for only one to two hours; so if you have a long labor, your spinal block may not last
Pudendal block A numbing medicine injected into the pudendal nerve through the vagina	Offers some pain relief without affecting your ability to push	Can be used only at the very end of delivery, when the baby's head is coming out

MONITORING YOUR BABY'S HEART RATE

During labor, your provider may want to check your baby's condition by monitoring his or her heart rate. This is called fetal monitoring, and there are several ways to do it:

- **An electronic fetal monitor.** Two monitors are fastened to your belly. One records your baby's heart rate; the other measures your contraction length and frequency.

- **A Doppler fetal monitor.** This is a small, handheld device that your provider presses against your belly to measure your baby's heart rate.

- **An electrode.** A thin wire (electrode) is inserted through the cervix and attached to your baby's scalp. The wire measures and records your baby's heart rate continuously on a bedside monitor.

If fetal heart rate monitoring through any of these means suggests that your baby is having a problem, your provider does other tests to find out more. An unborn baby's heart rate is usually around 120 to 160 beats per minute. If it slows down to 60 or 70 beats per minute (a situation called bradycardia), your provider suggests steps to bring it up to normal, such as having you change position, giving you intravenous fluids, and having you breathe in oxygen through a nose tube or mask.

ENTERING LABOR

When your labor contractions are strong and regular and your cervix has started to open, you are "in labor." There are three stages of labor.

Stage 1: Contractions

The first stage of labor has three parts: *early labor, active labor,* and *transition.*

During *early labor,* the powerful muscles in your uterus begin contracting, which causes your cervix to thin (efface) and dilate (open up). When the cervix is thinned and dilated to make an opening that is 10 centimeters in diameter (approximately four inches, or the width of a medium doughnut), your baby can pass from the uterus into the vagina on its way to the outside world. Dilation and effacement occur in early labor, during which time your contractions come every 5 to 20 minutes and last 30 to 60 seconds. Early labor can last anywhere from a few hours to a couple of days.

Most women can stay at home during early labor if their membranes are intact. Contractions can be strong but they are bearable, and there is time between contractions to rest, sleep, walk, watch TV, read, take a shower, or

> **Q:** *I'm worried—is there any chance I will lose control of my bowels or bladder while I'm pushing my baby out?*
>
> **A:** *You may lose control, but don't worry. Passing urine, gas, or stool is very common during delivery. Providers and delivery nurses think nothing of it because it happens so frequently, and there's no need to be embarrassed.*

relax with friends and family. If you're feeling uncomfortable, applying ice packs and massaging the lower back can provide relief. Be sure to drink water to keep yourself well hydrated for labor. And unless advised otherwise, continue to eat light meals and snacks throughout early labor so you're not starving during delivery. If possible, get some rest: your body has a lot of work ahead.

Early labor progresses to active labor when the cervix is dilated to 4 centimeters.

When you are in *active labor*, it's time to go to the hospital or birthing center. There, your provider examines your cervix, your baby's position, and your baby's location in the birth canal (called the station). You are also monitored to assess your baby's heartbeat, which can tell your provider how your baby is doing, and the contraction pattern, which shows the strength and frequency of the contractions.

During this part of labor, your contractions come more often (every two to five minutes), last longer (up to a minute), and get stronger. The amount of rest time between contractions gets smaller and smaller, giving you less and less recovery time between contractions. Your cervix continues to dilate, getting closer and closer to 10 centimeters. Active labor can last anywhere from a couple of hours to six hours. The rule of thumb is that you should dilate about 1 centimeter per hour during active labor. If this doesn't happen, your provider will evaluate your labor to see if you need additional medications to stimulate labor, or a c-section.

This is the time to use the relaxation and breathing techniques you learned during your childbirth classes. Your partner can help relieve your discomfort by massaging your shoulders and back or applying cold washcloths to your face. Keep in mind, though, that this kind of touching is not relaxing to some women. Changing positions, taking a bath, or going for brief walks can also help reduce pain. This is the time when you can consider getting epidural anesthesia, usually referred to simply as "an epidural," for pain relief.

The last part of active labor, when your cervix is dilated from 8 to 10 centimeters, is often called *transition*. During transition, contractions are strong and regular. Transition lasts from half an hour to two hours. When your cervix is fully open to 10 centimeters, you are considered "fully dilated." The first stage of labor ends, and it's time to push.

Stage 2: Birth

As stage 2 begins, your cervix is fully dilated and your contractions have pushed your baby far down into your pelvis. Your baby is ready to be born, and now you get to help by actively pushing along with each contraction in order to deliver your baby. You know when you're entering stage 2 because you start to have a strong urge to push.

Your provider and your labor nurse guide you through this stage, helping you to know when to push. When each contraction starts, you bear down and push as if you were having a bowel movement. Push as hard as you can for the length of the contraction. When the contraction lets up a bit, stop pushing and rest for a few seconds.

The second stage of labor is much faster than the first, typically lasting 20 minutes to 2 hours, and occasionally even longer.

Changing positions during this stage of labor can sometimes help you push more effectively. Sitting or squatting may make pushing easier and contractions less painful. If you've had an epidural, or if your baby is hooked up to a fetal monitor, you may be limited in what positions you can try.

Eventually your baby's head crowns (becomes visible to your provider). That means your baby is ready to be born.

If your baby can't come out easily, you may need an episiotomy or an assisted delivery. An episiotomy is a surgical cut in the perineum, the tissue between your vagina and your rectum. Assisted delivery is a delivery performed with the assistance of a medical instrument known as forceps (tongs) or by vacuum suction (using a suction cup attached to the baby's head). Babies delivered with forceps or vacuum suction may develop bruises or blisters on the scalp, but those are temporary.

When your baby is born, your provider suctions his or her mouth to remove secretions, which will help him or her begin breathing. The umbilical cord is clamped in two places by your provider and then cut in between, sometimes by your birth partner.

Q: *Will I have to have an episiotomy?*

A: *Episiotomies used to be fairly common. In recent years, however, research has shown that episiotomies are often not necessary, and episiotomy rates have gone down to fewer than 10 percent of births. If the perineum looks as if it will tear, your provider may choose to cut a small episiotomy with the rationale that a small, neat cut can be repaired and will heal more easily than a large tear. But either way, your perineum is very forgiving and heals within a few weeks.*

One minute after birth, your baby's vital signs are checked, and he or she receives what's called an Apgar score. Your provider gives a score between 0 and 2 for each of five things (skin color, heart rate, reflexes, muscle tone, and breathing rate) and adds them up. Babies with an Apgar score of 7 or above are usually fine; those with lower scores may need some extra care. The test is repeated after five minutes.

When you and your baby are ready, the delivery nurse places your baby on your chest or in your arms. This is your first chance to get to know your baby and start to fall in love face-to-face. If your baby is awake, this is a great time to put him or her to your breast to start the breastfeeding and bonding process. Sucking sends signals to your body to start to make breast milk.

You did it! The birth journey has come to an end and a whole new life awaits.

Stage 3: Afterbirth

The third stage of labor is the shortest. After your baby is born, you may continue to have mild contractions for 5 to 30 minutes. These contractions help separate the placenta (at this stage also called the afterbirth) from the uterus and help push it out. Your provider massages your uterus and with a gentle pull delivers the placenta. Because the placenta is very soft, women don't usually feel much when it is delivered. After the placenta comes out, your provider checks your uterus and may continue to massage it to make sure it is contracting down in size and the bleeding is stopping.

If you had an episiotomy, your provider stitches it up (using a local anesthetic injected with a tiny needle).

GIVING BIRTH BY ANOTHER ROUTE: CESAREAN SECTION

A cesarean section (c-section) is a surgical procedure used to deliver a baby through the mother's belly rather than her vagina. Although a c-section is major surgery, in situations when it is medically necessary it is safer for a mother and/or baby than a vaginal birth.

A c-section may be planned in advance when you and your provider know about a health problem that requires it—for example, if you are pregnant with triplets or are experiencing a complication such as placenta previa (where vaginal delivery would be too risky due to bleeding).

More often, c-sections are not planned; rather, they are determined to be necessary after a situation develops during a vaginal delivery—for example, your labor slows down or stops, or your baby's heart rate falls because he or she isn't getting enough oxygen.

A c-section does have some risks. For the mother, there is a chance of infection, adverse reactions to the anesthesia, blood clots that cause complications, excess bleeding, and injury to the bladder or bowel. It takes longer for the mother to recover from a c-section than a vaginal birth: a c-section typically requires a three- to four-day hospital stay rather than the usual two-day stay. Despite these risks, the benefits outweigh the risks in many cases when c-sections are needed.

Babies born by c-section are usually healthy. However, the surgery does increase the risk of certain side effects in babies, such as breathing problems. In addition, the anesthesia given to the mother can make a baby sluggish, which can interfere with early breastfeeding.

When a c-section is medically necessary, it can protect the health—and sometimes the life—of a mother and her baby. In these cases, the benefits of a c-section clearly outweigh its risks.

Some of the medical reasons for a c-section include:

- The mother is giving birth to more than one baby, or to a baby that is too big for a safe vaginal birth.

- Problems develop with the placenta or the umbilical cord.

- There are problems with the baby's position—for example, if the baby is breech (bottom-first rather than head-first) or the baby is in the transverse position (that is, the baby's shoulder enters the birth canal before the head).

- The baby is in distress (the heart rate is too low, for example) and needs to be delivered quickly.

- Labor slows down or stops.

- The mother has had a previous c-section or uterine surgery.

- Complications such as high blood pressure develop in the mother.

- Certain infections are present in the mother, such as active herpes at the time of delivery, which can be passed to the baby as it moves through the vagina at delivery.

- The baby is known to have certain kinds of birth defects.

If You Have a C-Section

Here's what you can expect during a c-section:

A nurse prepares you for surgery by washing your belly and, possibly, clipping or shaving the top part of your pubic hair. An intravenous (IV) line is inserted into a vein in your arm or hand, making it easy for your provider to give you fluids and medication. You are hooked up to machines that monitor your heart rate, blood pressure, and breathing, and a catheter is inserted into your bladder to drain urine during surgery. Once these things are done, an anesthesiologist gives you an epidural block, spinal block, or (less often) general anesthesia.

In the operating room, your provider makes a cut of about six inches in your skin at your bikini line, just above the pubic hairline. Then your provider cuts through the fat below your skin and separates your abdominal muscles in the middle. A cut is made toward the bottom of the uterus, and the uterus is opened. The baby is lifted, or delivered, through that opening.

If the baby has to come out in a hurry—like in about one minute—your provider may make a vertical cut from the navel to the pubic bone and a vertical incision in the uterus. This leaves a more prominent scar, but it's faster than the bikini-line cut. A vertical incision in the uterus has a higher likelihood than a bikini-line cut of pulling apart during future labors, so when it's used, it usually means future babies will need to be delivered by c-section rather than vaginally.

Once your baby is delivered and the umbilical cord is cut, your provider removes the placenta and closes the incisions—both uterine and abdominal—using suture material on the inside and surgical staples on the skin. The entire procedure takes about 45 to 60 minutes.

After surgery, you are taken to the recovery room, where you are monitored to make sure you are recovering properly. Then you are transferred to a hospital room.

C-Section by Choice: A Healthy Decision?

C-section rates in the United States have risen dramatically during the past few decades. Today, one in three babies is born by c-section. Having a c-section adds some risk factors to future pregnancies, however. Once you've had a c-section, it's more difficult to give birth vaginally in the future because of a higher risk of serious complications such as placenta problems and uterine rupture. With each c-section you have, chances of complications increase. These risks are worth taking when c-section is medically necessary. But without medical reason, risks outweigh benefits.

Although the decision to do a c-section should be made by a woman and her provider, the March of Dimes advises against elective c-sections—those that are not medically necessary—especially before 39 completed weeks of pregnancy.

IN DEPTH

Vaginal Birth After C-Section

See page 259

WHEN YOUR BABY IS OVERDUE

The average healthy pregnancy is 40 weeks. Just as some pregnancies result in premature birth, some pregnant mothers go *past* their due date. While it is unusual, a pregnancy that lasts longer than 42 weeks is called a post-term pregnancy.

Although many post-term babies are healthy, some risks do start to increase after 41 to 42 weeks. An overdue pregnancy takes a toll on the placenta, amniotic fluid, and umbilical cord. As the baby grows larger, the chances of stillbirth and delivery injuries go up, and there is a greater likelihood that the baby will experience meconium aspiration (inhaling stool from the amniotic fluid into the lungs) or a condition called dysmaturity syndrome (in which the baby is no longer getting enough nourishment because the placenta is aging and becoming calcified).

When a baby is overdue, the provider may do some tests to check on the baby's health. They include:

- ■ *Ultrasound exam*

- ■ *Kick count,* which is a count of how many times your baby moves or kicks you during a certain period of time

Q: *What is a "kick count," and when is it done?*

A: *Beginning at about week 28, your provider may ask you to do a kick count. (Some providers recommend this for all of their patients; others advise it only if a problem is suspected.) This requires a dedicated time when you pay attention to your baby's kicks, turns, twists, rolls, and jabs. Typically a baby moves 10 times in less than two hours. Select a time of day when your baby is usually active, and do the kick count at roughly that same time each day. If the baby has fewer than 10 kicks in two hours, or if there's a significant decrease in fetal movement, call your health-care provider, who may recommend tests such as an ultrasound to check on the baby's health. Feeling fewer kicks than expected doesn't necessarily mean there's something wrong with your baby, but if the kick count is low, it's a good idea to have it checked out.*

- **Nonstress test,** in which a fetal monitor measures your baby's heart rate for a certain amount of time

- **Biophysical profile,** which uses a fetal monitor and an ultrasound to score a baby on each of five factors (nonstress test, body movements, breathing movements, muscle tone, and the amount of amniotic fluid)

- **Contraction stress test,** which compares your baby's heart rate at rest with the heart rate during contractions induced by a shot of oxytocin or by nipple stimulation

If these tests suggest that your baby is in good condition, you can continue to wait for labor to begin naturally. If they raise concerns, your provider may wish to induce labor or perform a c-section. Providers rarely allow a pregnancy to go beyond 42 weeks.

Chapter Thirteen

Healthy Baby

Babies are not necessarily beautiful when they emerge from the birth canal. They are likely to be wrinkled, wet, bloody, and blotchy. They may be covered with a waxy white coating (called vernix caseosa) and may have swollen eyelids and genitals, a misshapen head, white pimples on the face (called milia), and soft, furry hair (called lanugo) on the face, shoulders, and back. Don't worry, this is all normal. Babies look better after the delivery nurse cleans them up.

While you deliver the placenta and get stitches to close up your episiotomy (if you had one), your delivery nurse measures and weighs your baby, cleans the fluids off your baby's skin, applies eye ointment to prevent infection, and uses nontoxic ink to take your baby's footprints. Your baby also receives a vitamin K shot in the thigh, which is needed for blood clotting, and a hepatitis B vaccine.

You, your partner, and your baby receive matching bracelets for security purposes, usually before your baby leaves your side. After the initial cleaning and shots, your baby is given a hat and is wrapped in a blanket. Newborns need to stay warm; in fact, sometimes they are placed under a heat lamp for extra warmth.

If your baby needs special care—for example, if your baby has trouble breathing, is premature (born before 37 completed weeks), is too small, or is sick—a nurse takes him or her from the delivery room to the nursery. If a baby has critical medical needs that go beyond what can be provided in the delivery hospital's nursery, the baby's provider may recommend transporting the baby to a neonatal intensive care unit (NICU—pronounced *nick*-you) at another hospital. NICUs have highly trained staff and advanced medical equipment to provide 24/7 critical care to newborns.

NEWBORN SCREENING

In the hospital, babies receive tests that are referred to as newborn screening. These tests are very important.

Most babies are born healthy. Some, though, do have health problems. And sometimes those problems are not visible. A baby can be born with a health problem but not show any signs of the problem at first.

Newborn screening can help uncover those hidden health problems. When they're found early, such problems can be treated early—often making it possible to avoid more serious health conditions as the baby grows up.

Newborn screening checks for serious but rare conditions at birth. It includes blood, hearing, and heart screening. Newborn screening checks to see if your baby is more likely than other babies to have particular health problems.

Most newborn screening (except for hearing and heart) is done with a blood test. During the blood test, one of the nurses in the nursery pricks your baby's heel with a needle to get just a few drops of blood for testing. The hospital sends the blood to a state lab for testing. The lab then sends the results back to your baby's health-care provider.

There are two different tests that can check your baby's hearing and how he or she responds to sounds. These tests, which are done in the nursery at the hospital, use either a tiny, soft earphone or a microphone placed in your baby's ear.

Babies are also screened for a heart condition called critical congenital heart disease (CCHD) using a painless test called pulse oximetry. This test checks the amount of oxygen in your baby's blood by using a sensor that's usually attached to the baby's finger or foot. If the test shows low oxygen levels, your baby needs more tests to check for CCHD.

If newborn screening results aren't normal, it doesn't mean for sure that your baby has a health problem. It simply means that your baby needs more testing. Your baby's provider will then recommend another kind of test, called a diagnostic test, to see if there truly is a health problem.

The March of Dimes recommends that all babies be screened for at least 31 health conditions. Each of these health problems can be treated effectively if found early. However, each state has its own rules about how many health conditions are checked with newborn screening.

All states require newborn screening for at least 26 health conditions. Some states require screening for additional conditions—even up to 50 or more. You can ask your health-care provider how many conditions your state requires testing for. Alternatively, contact your state health department or the National Newborn Screening and Genetics Resource Center (http://genes-r-us.uthscsa.edu/).

THE CIRCUMCISION DECISION

Circumcision is the surgical removal of a boy's foreskin (the fold of skin that covers the tip of the penis at birth). Circumcision is a parental choice. Not all boys are circumcised.

You and your partner can decide what's best for your son. You may choose circumcision because all the men in your family are circumcised. Or you may opt either for or against circumcision to follow religious or cultural traditions. You may choose not to have your son circumcised so that he doesn't have any medical risks from the surgery.

The American Academy of Pediatrics (AAP) says circumcision has health benefits that outweigh its risks. The organization says there's not enough scientific evidence of benefits to recommend circumcision for *all* boys, however. AAP encourages parents to make their decision after talking about the procedure with their health-care provider.

Circumcision does lower the risk of urinary tract infections (UTIs), cancer of the penis, and certain STIs, including HIV/AIDS. However, UTIs are uncommon in boys, penile cancer is rare, and there are more effective ways to prevent STIs.

There is also a small risk of infection and bleeding, and in rare cases there can be injury to the penis, with resultant scarring. But circumcised babies usually get through the procedure without any problem, and the site heals in 7 to 10 days.

Your provider may use a cream anesthetic or a shot of anesthesia to reduce any pain your baby feels. Even with these methods, babies often cry during circumcision and for a short time after it.

Circumcisions are typically done in the hospital before you and your baby are discharged. Some baby boys are circumcised in the first days of life at home, as part of a religious or cultural tradition.

CARING FOR YOUR BABY

Healthy babies and mothers usually stay in the hospital for two nights before being discharged. This brief lull is a good time to start learning about how to care for your baby. The nurses can answer your questions about diapering, bathing, swaddling, dressing, feeding, and burping your baby. They will also show you how to care for your baby's umbilical cord stump and circumcision

For Parents of Preemies

Babies born early—before 37 completed weeks of pregnancy—usually have to spend some time in the nursery or NICU. Having a premature baby can feel overwhelming, especially if your baby requires extensive medical care.

We don't know all the reasons babies are born prematurely, though research is bringing us closer to finding the answers. You may be wondering why you went into labor early and whether there is anything you can do differently if you decide to get pregnant again. You may feel you have a lot to learn about premature birth and preemies, whether your baby was born just a couple of weeks early, or months too soon.

Many people feel changed by the experience of having a baby prematurely. Connecting with other parents who have been through similar experiences can help. Some parents find that telling their own story and helping others helps them understand and cope with their own experience.

You can learn more and connect with other parents of premature babies on the March of Dimes websites: marchofdimes.com, nacersano.org, and marchofdimes.com/shareyourstory.

Q: What is jaundice?

A: *Jaundice, a condition in which a baby's skin becomes tinged with yellow, is common in newborns. It is caused by a buildup of bilirubin, a blood by-product that is removed from the body by the liver. Sometimes a baby's liver doesn't do a good job of removing bilirubin during the first few days of life. Having jaundice doesn't mean your baby has a liver problem— it just means the liver needs a little extra time after birth to get up to speed. Although jaundice is not serious, if it becomes excessive and is not treated, it can lead to brain damage. A baby with jaundice needs to be seen by a provider and sometimes must receive care in the hospital. Some babies with jaundice need phototherapy, a treatment in which they are placed under lights that aid the excretion of bilirubin.*

site (if you had a boy who was circumcised). Most hospitals have a lactation nurse available to give breastfeeding advice.

After babies are born, they are cared for by their own provider—a pediatrician, a family physician, or a pediatric nurse-practitioner. Ideally you will have already chosen your pediatric provider during your pregnancy.

If the pediatric provider you chose is associated with the hospital where you gave birth, the provider sees your baby in the hospital. If that provider is not available, a hospital pediatrician examines your baby after delivery, and your provider takes over your baby's care after discharge from the hospital.

When you leave the hospital, you receive information about when to schedule your baby's first appointment. Ask for a copy of your baby's medical record to take with you if your pediatric provider doesn't have access to it through the hospital's computer system.

PROTECTING YOUR BABY FROM SIDS

Sudden infant death syndrome (SIDS) is the sudden, unexplained death of an infant during the first year of life. It can occur without warning in a baby who appears healthy. It is most likely to happen when a baby between the ages of two months and four months is sleeping. It's sometimes called crib death. Sadly, thousands of babies die of SIDS in the United States each year.

Researchers don't know why SIDS occurs. However, they have identified a list of factors that are linked to an increased risk of SIDS:

- Sleeping on the tummy or side

- Sleeping with another person—half of all SIDS cases occur when babies are sleeping with a parent or caretaker in a bed, on a sofa, or on a chair

- Sleeping with blankets, electric blankets, pillows, sleep positioners, or other soft bedding that can interfere with the baby's breathing

- Having ongoing exposure to secondhand smoke

- Having a teen mother

- Having a mother who had poor prenatal care during pregnancy

- Having a parent who smokes, drinks alcohol, or uses street drugs

- Becoming overheated while sleeping

- Being a boy

- Being an African American or Native American

- Being a multiple (such as a twin or triplet), or having been conceived soon after the birth of a sibling

- Being formula-fed—being breastfed reduces colds and other mild infections, which can increase SIDS risk

- Having a sibling who had SIDS (possibly)

- Being a preemie or having been born with a low birthweight

- Having certain genetic factors that raise risk

- Living in poverty

You can't change some SIDS risk factors, such as being a boy or a twin. But there are lots of things you *can* change—avoiding having secondhand smoke in your home, for example, or making sure there is no soft bedding or any object but the mattress and the baby in your baby's crib. By taking steps to make your baby's sleeping environment as safe as possible, you can lower your baby's risk of SIDS.

Always place your baby on his back to sleep—even during naps. Babies who sleep on their backs, rather than their sides or their tummies, have a lower risk of SIDS. Make sure all your baby's caretakers know this.

When to Call Your Baby's Provider

Call your baby's provider right away if your baby has:

- A change in the way he holds his body—for example, if he seems floppy or lethargic
- A persistent cough
- A rectal temperature over 100.4°F or under 97.8°F
- A seizure or unusual shaking
- A sudden lack of interest in feeding
- An episode of vomiting (not merely spitting up) more than two or three times in one day
- Blood in the vomit or stool, or coming from the nose
- Blue lips or fingernails
- Diarrhea
- Difficulty waking up or unusual sleepiness
- Few or no stools
- Fewer than four wet diapers in 24 hours
- Pus, discharge, warmth, bleeding, or redness at the umbilical cord stump or circumcision site
- Trouble breathing or unusual breathing—for example, gasping, wheezing, or making whistling sounds while breathing
- Unusual crying spells or crying that can't be consoled
- Yellow or green mucus in the eyes
- Yellowish skin or eyes

If you're not sure whether to call your baby's provider, don't sit and worry—make the call. Pediatricians and other child-care providers expect frequent calls from new parents. Follow your instincts.

Q: *Sleeping with a blanket is linked to SIDS risk—but I don't want my baby to be cold. How can I keep my baby warm?*

A: *Your baby should be fine dressed in footie pajamas or a sleep sack, which are much safer than blankets. (Choose warmer sleepers if your baby is due in the winter, and lighter ones for summer.) Keep the room temperature warm enough for an adult to sleep comfortably—but not too warm, because overheating during sleep has also been linked to SIDS.*

SHIELDING YOUR BABY FROM SECONDHAND SMOKE

When someone in your home smokes, your baby smokes. This is called secondhand smoking or involuntary smoking. Exhaled smoke (along with the smoke created by the burning of a cigarette, cigar, or pipe) fills the air in your home. When babies breathe, they pull the smoke—and the 50 cancer-causing chemicals it contains—into their tiny lungs.

Babies exposed to secondhand smoke have an increased risk of SIDS, ear infections, colds, pneumonia, bronchitis, severe asthma, headaches, sore throats, dizziness, nausea, lack of energy, and fussiness.

Later in life, children who live with smokers have a higher risk of tooth decay, poor lung development, lung cancer, heart disease, and cataracts.

There are so many great reasons to quit smoking—and having a new baby is among the best. Don't let anyone in your home or near your baby smoke.

Chapter Fourteen

Baby Mealtime

Other than sleeping, your newborn spends more time feeding than doing anything else during the first few months of life. A baby's body grows and develops rapidly—most newborns double their birthweight by six months of age, and triple it by the time they're a year old. In order for babies to grow at that rate and thrive, they need food that meets all of their nutritional needs.

Breast milk is the best food for babies. The March of Dimes joins with the American Academy of Pediatrics (AAP) in encouraging all mothers to breast-feed if they are able. The AAP, America's number one authority on children's health, recommends exclusive breastfeeding for six months.

If breast milk is not an option, babies should be fed infant formula that is appropriate for their needs.

Whether you feed your baby breast milk or formula, you probably have a lot of questions. This chapter answers your questions. It also provides resources for moms who need some extra help feeding their babies.

WHY BREAST MILK?

Breast milk is perfectly designed for your baby. It contains all of the protein, carbohydrates, fat, vitamins, minerals, and water your baby needs; and as your baby's nutritional needs change, so does your breast milk. It has antibodies from your body that help your baby's body fight infection, and fatty acids such as DHA that help your baby's brain develop.

Your body has an amazing ability to manufacture breast milk to meet your baby's specific needs. For example, if your baby is born prematurely, your breast milk is different than it would be if your baby were born full term, because a premature baby's nutritional needs differ from a full-term baby's. When your baby has growth spurts, your body responds by boosting its production of breast milk.

During the first few days of your baby's life, your breasts produce a sticky, yellowish kind of milk called colostrum. This early milk is high in protein and immune substances that your baby needs early in life. After a few days your milk becomes thinner and more milky-looking. Its fat and protein content change as your baby's needs for these nutrients change.

Breast milk offers a long list of benefits. Compared with formula-fed babies, babies who are breastfed have a lower rate of allergies, colds, pneumonia, bronchitis, constipation, diabetes, infections, and gas; in addition, they have lower rates of sudden infant death syndrome (SIDS). Children and adults who were breastfed are less likely to become overweight or obese or to develop diabetes.

Breastfeeding benefits moms. They have less postpartum bleeding, because the hormones released during early breastfeeding help the uterus to contract. What's more, they return to their preconception weight faster than those who don't breastfeed.

There's a financial bonus to breastfeeding, too: breastfeeding exclusively can save new parents up to $1,000 in their baby's first year on formula and bottles.

LEARNING TO BREASTFEED

Breastfeeding is a completely natural process, but that doesn't mean it always comes naturally to moms or babies. Breastfeeding is a *learned* skill. Not surprisingly, then, you and your baby may need some help getting the hang of breastfeeding. Fortunately, help is available.

Take time before your baby is born to educate the people around you about the benefits of breastfeeding. Your partner, your mother, and other family members may not understand why you're choosing to breastfeed. In past generations, new mothers were sometimes told that formula is better for babies than breast milk. Most health-care providers now know that is not true, but it's a myth that some people—especially older women who were told not to bother breastfeeding their babies—still believe.

In the hospital, start breastfeeding your baby within an hour of birth. Be sure to tell the nurses beforehand that you want to breastfeed and don't want them to give your baby any formula. If you're having any trouble breastfeeding, ask your provider or nurse for help. Many hospitals employ lactation consultants—nurses who specialize in helping women with breastfeeding. Working with a lactation consultant in the hospital can help get you and your baby off to a great start.

After you take your baby home, call your baby's provider if you're having trouble breastfeeding. Pediatricians and family-care providers sometimes have lactation nurses on staff, or they can recommend independent lactation consultants in your area. Look for a certified lactation counselor (CLC), certified by the Healthy Children's Center for Breastfeeding, or a lactation consultant certified by the International Board of Lactation Consultant Examiners (IBLCE).

Another great source of breastfeeding support is La Leche League International, a nonprofit organization dedicated to providing education, information, support, and encouragement to women who want to breastfeed. La Leche offers group meetings and breastfeeding help from local leaders throughout the United States and the world. To find out more, go to the La Leche website (www.lllusa.org) or call (877) 4-LALECHE (452-5324).

BREASTFEEDING Q&A

New moms usually have a lot of questions about breastfeeding. Here are answers to the ones that are most commonly asked:

Q: *Who should not breastfeed?*

A: It's not safe for women to breastfeed if:
- They have active herpes sores on their breasts.
- They have HIV/AIDS or active tuberculosis.
- They drink alcohol or take street drugs.
- They take certain medications that can pass through the milk and harm a baby.

- They've had certain kinds of breast surgery—although many women who have had breast surgery can breastfeed successfully. Women with nipple piercings and tattoos may also be able to breastfeed.

Q: *Can moms breastfeed babies in the NICU?*

A: Moms who have very small, sick, or premature babies in the NICU may not be able to breastfeed their babies. However, they can usually feed them *expressed* breast milk with a specially designed feeding tube or dropper.

Q: *Can women with flat or inverted nipples breastfeed?*

A: Usually they can. Milk comes from the areola, the area around the nipple, so women with inverted or flat nipples can usually breastfeed successfully. Wearing plastic breast shells inside your bra may help draw out inverted or flat nipples. Talk with your provider about your concerns or meet with a lactation consultant for support.

Q: *Does breastfeeding hurt?*

A: It can cause some discomfort at first, but that shouldn't last more than a few days. If it actually *hurts,* your baby may be latching on incorrectly, taking just the nipple into his mouth instead of the areola around the nipple. Or you may have an infection in your breast that requires treatment. Contact your provider if you feel soreness or pain while your baby breastfeeds, or if your nipples are cracked or bleeding.

Q: *Do breastfeeding babies need any extra food or liquids?*

A: During the first six months, breast milk alone is fine for babies with no special medical needs. Your breastfeeding baby doesn't need water and should never have cow's milk, fruit juice, sugar water, cereal, or any other drink or food. When your baby is about six months old, his or her provider will probably suggest that you start introducing solid foods; but until then, all your baby needs is breast milk.

Q: *Do breastfeeding babies need to take any supplements?*

A: The March of Dimes recommends that all breastfed babies and some formula-fed babies receive vitamin D drops (400 IU per day). Check with your baby's provider to make sure vitamin D drops are right for your baby. Vitamin D drops are available over the counter at drugstores and pharmacies. When you use them, make sure to fill the dropper to exactly 400 IU—no more and no less!

Q: *Should I change the way I eat while I'm breastfeeding?*

A: When you were pregnant, you needed an extra 300 calories a day. When you're breastfeeding, that number goes up to 500 calories. As during pregnancy, try to get all your extra calories from health-promoting foods such as lean meats, low-fat dairy foods, whole grains, fruits, vegetables, and legumes. You should also make sure to drink enough water. After all, you need to take in enough water for yourself and your baby. Aim to drink 8 to 12 glasses of water a day. Get in the habit of having a glass of water every time you sit down to breastfeed.

Q: *Should I continue to take my prenatal multivitamins while I'm breastfeeding?*

A: Yes. It's not a bad idea to continue taking your prenatal vitamins until you run out, and then switch to a regular daily multivitamin. Your provider or your baby's provider may recommend additional supplements if you or your baby has special needs. For example, if you're a vegetarian, your provider will want to be sure you're getting enough vitamin B_{12}, which can be in short supply in women who don't eat animal foods. A shortage of vitamin B_{12} in a mother's diet can contribute to brain development problems in a breastfeeding baby.

Q: *Can I take medicines while breastfeeding?*

A: Many drugs are safe to take during breastfeeding, but a few are not. Check with your provider before taking any medicine, including prescription and over-the-counter drugs, as well as herbs and other natural remedies.

Q: *How long should I breastfeed?*

A: The American Academy of Pediatrics recommends breastfeeding for one year, if possible (and giving *only* breast milk for the first six months)—or as long as you and your baby desire. Breastfeeding for a full year is good for your baby, but it's not possible for every woman. Try to breastfeed as long as you can—and remember, no matter how long you breastfeed, your baby is benefiting.

Q: *How often do I breastfeed my newborn?*

A: Breastfeed whenever your baby is hungry. For a newborn, that's every two to three hours, 8 to 12 times a day. Your baby may feed even more often during growth spurts, which typically occur at the ages of two weeks, six weeks, three months, and six months. As babies get bigger, they need to feed less often.

Q: *Do I need to use birth control while I'm breastfeeding?*

A: Yes. Even though breastfeeding women sometimes have delayed periods, they may still get pregnant if they are having unprotected sex. Talk with your provider about what kind of birth control is best for you.

Q: *How do I hold my baby while breastfeeding?*

A: Sit up and hold your baby in your arms with baby's head in the crook of your elbow and baby's tummy facing your tummy. This is called the cradle hold. Use a pillow on your lap to help support your baby. Cup your breast (the one on the same side as your baby's head) and tickle baby's lip with your nipple. When your baby opens his or her mouth, firmly bring your baby to your breast. Your baby has to have at least half an inch of your areola (the darker skin around the nipple) in his or her mouth to start milk flowing. Be sure not to push the baby's cheek away from your breast inadvertently— babies naturally move toward the side that's touched.

Alternately, hold your baby tucked under your arm (like a football) with your baby's belly against your side. Support your baby's head with your hand (right hand for right-breast feeding, left for left) and guide your nipple to your baby's mouth with the other hand. This is called the football hold.

Q: *I'm going back to work. Can I still breastfeed my baby?*

A: Yes. When you're at work, you can collect (express) milk with a breast pump and store it in a refrigerator or freezer. Your child-care provider can feed expressed milk to your baby with a bottle. When you're not at work, you can continue to breastfeed your baby as usual.

Q: *Do I need a breast pump?*

A: Having a breast pump is *necessary* for working moms who want to express milk and *handy* for moms who would like to give their baby an occasional bottle. Breast pumps come in a variety of styles and prices; you can also rent a pump. You also need bags or bottles to store expressed milk in. Ask your provider, lactation consultant, or hospital staff for information about buying or renting pumps. (If you rent, you'll still have to buy new accessories such as tubing, bags, bottles, and nipples.) Working moms usually need to pump (express) their milk two or three times a day. For them, an electric double-pump is the fastest way to empty both breasts at work.

Q: *How long can I store breast milk for future use?*

A: Breast milk can be refrigerated for up to eight days in a refrigerator with a temperature of 32 to 39 degrees. (A small refrigerator thermometer can tell you how cold your refrigerator is.) Breast milk can also be stored for up to three months in a freezer that has a separate door, or two weeks in a freezer compartment that's located inside a refrigerator. To defrost breast milk, run it under warm water or place it in a bowl of warm water. Smell or taste it before feeding it to your baby to make sure it hasn't gone bad.

Q: *How do I know when my baby is hungry or full?*

A: Some signs of hunger include rooting (searching for the breast), showing increased alertness or activity, puckering the mouth, and sucking on fingers or a fist. A baby who is very hungry starts to cry, but it's best not to wait for crying because a crying baby may be too upset to latch on to the breast. Your baby feeds until his or her hunger is appeased—usually for about 10 to 15 minutes on each breast. Signs of fullness include turning away from the breast, sealing his or her lips, spitting out the nipple, losing interest in the nipple, and getting sleepy. Once your baby is full, don't try to push him or her to eat more.

Q: *How do I know my baby is eating enough?*

A: A well-fed baby looks happy and satisfied, gains an adequate amount of weight, has six to eight wet diapers a day, and has two to five stools a day.

FORMULA FEEDING

Women who don't breastfeed—either by choice or by circumstance—can feed their babies formula. Baby formula is designed to be as close as possible to human breast milk.

There are several kinds of baby formula. Ready-to-use formula is the most convenient, because it requires no mixing with water. Convenience comes at a price, however: ready-to-use formula is more expensive than other formula. Concentrated liquid formula is a liquid that must be mixed with water. Powdered formula is a powder that must be mixed with water. Powdered formula is the least-expensive option.

Iron-fortified formula, which is available in both ready-to-use and add-water versions, is recommended for most babies, because babies' iron stores tend to be low.

Cow's milk formula is recommended for most babies. It is processed in such a way that its proteins closely resemble the proteins in human breast milk. Although cow's milk formula is safe for babies, *actual* cow's milk should never be fed to babies before they are a year old. Never give your baby homemade formula made from cow's milk, goat's milk, or evaporated/condensed milk.

Soy formula, as its name suggests, is made from soy rather than cow's milk. Soy formula is recommended for babies who have a milk allergy or intolerance.

There are various kinds of formula for babies who can't have either cow's milk formula or soy formula. Protein hydrolysate formula is for infants who have allergies or can't tolerate other kinds of formula. Lactose-free formula is for babies who can't digest lactose, a sugar in milk. (Lactose intolerance can cause gas, belly pain, and other symptoms.) Specialty formulas are available for premature babies, low birthweight babies, and babies with certain medical problems (including reflux). Your baby's provider must write a prescription for medically necessary specialty formulas, which are usually expensive but may be covered by health insurance.

Preparing Formula Safely

In the kitchen, formula can become contaminated with germs if it's not prepared and handled correctly. You can keep your baby's formula safe by following these prep steps:

- Wash your hands well before working with formula.

- Sterilize bottles and nipples before using them the first time by boiling them in water for 5 to 10 minutes. If bottles have been used before, wash them in hot, soapy water and rinse them well—or wash them in a dishwasher.

- Rinse the top of the can with hot water, if that's how your formula is packaged.

- Follow the preparation directions on the formula package exactly. Measure water and formula carefully using marked measuring cups or spoons that have been washed in hot, soapy water and rinsed well.

- Don't add anything else to formula, such as sugar, rice cereal, or cow's milk.

- If you're making more formula than you need at the time, refrigerate what you don't use.

- Prepare formula with tap water if your home's tap water is free from lead and other contaminants described in chapter 8. If your tap water isn't safe, use bottled water. Be sure to let your provider know you're using bottled water. Most brands contain no fluoride, so your provider may recommend that you give your baby fluoride drops. If you use tap water that's not fluoridated, mention that to your provider as well.

- Feed the formula to your baby at room temperature or warmed up in a bowl of water. (Don't microwave formula, because it may get too hot in some spots and burn your baby's mouth.) Check the temperature of the formula before feeding.

- Talk with your baby's provider about how much formula to feed your baby. Most babies need about 2½ ounces per pound of body weight per day—but that's just a rough estimate. Follow your baby's hunger and fullness cues as well as your provider's recommendation.

- After feeding, discard any formula remaining in your baby's bottle.

INSIDE YOUR BABY'S DIAPERS

New parents are often surprised at what they find in their baby's diapers. A newborn's stool looks much different than the stool of an older baby, toddler, or child. New parents may also be surprised to learn that a newborn needs a diaper change as many as eight times a day. Every time your baby eats, his brain sends a signal to his digestive system to release urine and stool. But don't worry—feedings and diaper changes go down in number as your baby grows.

Just after birth, your baby's stools are loose, black, and sticky. After a day or two, the stools of breastfed babies turn loose and mustard-colored, and contain what look like small seeds; formula-fed babies have soft, tan stools. After about a week your baby's stools become slightly firmer.

Normal newborn stools can look like diarrhea, so if your baby actually has diarrhea, it can be hard to detect. A change in frequency or consistency of stools, an unusual smell, or blood in the stools can be a sign of diarrhea. If you're not sure whether your baby's stools are normal, call your baby's provider.

Chapter Fifteen

Back on Track

Your baby has arrived, but you're not quite finished with the physical changes of pregnancy. During the days and weeks after birth—called the postpartum period—your body heals and recuperates from the stresses of labor and delivery. Your breasts start to produce nutrient-rich milk for your baby. And you begin a lifetime of parenting.

Overall, it takes six to eight weeks for your body to return to normal. Two exceptions to this timeline are your breasts (if you're breastfeeding) and your weight, which may take longer to return to what it was before you got pregnant.

The postpartum period can be challenging. During this time, you're taking care of at least two people: your new baby and yourself. And if you have children at home—especially toddlers—they need your care and attention also. It can be tough to balance your baby's needs with your own, as well as those of other family members. You need help and support from your partner, family, and friends.

Emotionally, you experience many feelings during the postpartum period: joy that you've finally met the baby who has been growing inside of you for so long, relief that labor and delivery are over, anxiety if this is your first baby and you're not yet confident in your mothering skills, sadness if labor and delivery didn't go quite the way you planned—if you had hoped for a vaginal

Your postpartum body can seem bewildering. But knowing what to expect and how to ease some of the discomforts can make these weeks easier. Before you know it, you will feel like yourself again.

birth and needed a c-section, for example—and worry if you or your baby has any health problems. These feelings, and others, are all completely normal for new mothers.

Physically, there's your uterus, which had grown big enough to hold your baby and now gradually shrinks back down to the size of a pear. You no longer need the extra blood your body made while you were pregnant, so your body breaks it down. Some of the extra hair your body grew in response to the action of pregnancy hormones starts to fall out.

Your postpartum body can seem bewildering. But knowing what to expect and how to ease some of the discomforts can make these weeks easier. Before you know it, you will feel like yourself again.

RECOVERING FROM CHILDBIRTH

Here are some of the things you may be experiencing after you give birth, followed by suggestions on how to feel better:

Soreness in the perineum Your perineum—the area between your vagina and your rectum—stretches quite a bit during vaginal birth, which can lead to soreness after delivery. The area may feel even more uncomfortable if it tore or if you had an episiotomy (a cut made in the vaginal opening to make room for your baby to come through), both of which require stitches. There are a few ways to relieve perineal soreness:

- Apply an ice pack or ice wrapped in a towel to the area. If one of the nurses in the hospital doesn't offer you an ice pack, ask for one.

- Take a sitz bath by using just a few inches of water in the bathtub or by soaking your bottom in a basin. If you have stitches, don't wipe the area; instead, clean it by squirting it with warm water as needed using a device called a peri-bottle (which you can bring home from the hospital). Again, if one of the nurses doesn't offer it, ask.

- Take pressure off your perineum by sitting on a pillow or a round "dough-nut" cushion. Ask if your hospital provides such cushions to new mothers. If not, buy one in the pharmacy.

- When you're ready, start doing Kegel exercises (see page 65). They increase blood flow and strengthen pelvic muscles, both of which help the perineum heal.

Embarrassment over a belly that still looks pregnant It takes a while for your uterus to shrink down in size. The unfortunate result of this is that you may still look pregnant after you give birth. In fact, you may need to wear maternity clothes or loose clothes for a while. This is normal—although in our celebrity-crazed culture, you may feel that if you're not wearing size-2 jeans a few weeks after delivery, there's something wrong with you. Pay no attention to the ridiculous expectations set by the media for what a woman "should" look like after she gives birth. Expect your bump to stay around for a while.

Afterbirth pain In order for the uterus to return to its preconception size, its strong muscles contract. This can sometimes cause discomfort that's known as afterbirth pain. It can be especially intense while nursing: your baby's suck-ing tells your brain to release oxytocin, which causes the uterus to contract. Afterbirth pain should go away in a week or two.

Sweating New mothers are often surprised to find themselves sweating after delivery. Postpartum sweating, caused by hormone changes, may be accom-panied by chills or hot flashes. Know that these sensations are caused by your body adjusting to the end of the hormonal changes of pregnancy. You're not sick. Make yourself comfortable, and rest assured that your symptoms will go away within around six weeks of delivery.

Frequent urination Another way your body rids itself of fluids it no longer needs is through urination. Expect to make frequent trips to the bathroom for a few weeks.

Vaginal bleeding Some bleeding is normal for up to six weeks after birth as your body lets go of the contents of your uterus. This vaginal discharge is called lochia. During the first four or five days, the flow of bloody fluid is typically heavy and bright red. Over time the amount of blood lessens, and the color lightens from bright red to pink to brown to yellow. Use sanitary napkins (*not* tampons) to absorb the bloody fluid. The hospital will probably provide some superabsorbent pads. If there are any left at the end of your stay, take some with you when you leave. They're great for the first few days at home.

If bleeding is unusually heavy, it could be a sign that there's a problem with your uterus, vagina, or cervix. Sometimes, for example, a piece of the placenta remains in the uterus after birth. This can lead to an infection of the lining of the uterus (the endometrium) known as endometritis. Symptoms of infection include abnormal or foul-smelling vaginal discharge, backache, chills, fever, headache, or tenderness in your lower belly. If you experience any of these signs, be sure to call your provider. Endometritis can be treated with antibiotics after the placenta tissue is removed by D&C.

An increase in bleeding could also be a sign that you need to slow down, take it easy, and make sure your body has a chance to recover from the amazing experience of labor and delivery.

How do you know when you're bleeding too much? A little blood goes a long way in the toilet or on a white sheet, and it can be hard to know what's okay and what's not. If you're concerned—or if you start to feel weak or dizzy, the bleeding is getting heavier rather than lighter, or the bleeding is bright red rather than dark red/brown—call your provider.

Generally, it's a good idea to take showers instead of baths until your lochia stops. Soothe your bottom in a sitz bath as needed.

Blood clots It's normal for you to pass big globs of bloody material—blood clots—during the first week after birth. Don't be shocked by their size: they can be as big as golf balls.

Broken blood vessels in your face Using every ounce of strength in your body to push out your baby can cause some of the small blood vessels in your face to burst open, leaving your face with a road map of red lines. Don't worry—these tiny vessels usually repair themselves, and the redness goes down within six weeks.

Swollen breasts The first milk your breasts produce is a sticky, yellowish fluid called colostrum. This milk is high in protein and immune substances that your baby needs early in life—it's important that your baby get this valuable first milk. Two or three days after birth, your breasts begin to make a much larger amount of milk. When this happens, your breasts may swell up to a surprisingly large size. They may also become hard, lumpy, and either tender or downright painful. This is called engorgement. There are several ways to relieve engorgement:

- Breastfeed your baby frequently. Try not to wait until your breasts are fully engorged, because your baby may have trouble getting the nipple in his or her mouth. If this happens, expressing a small amount of milk (manually or with a breast pump) can make latching on easier. Avoid expressing more than a few drops of milk, however; if you do, it sends a message to your breasts to make even more milk.

- Wear a supportive nursing bra.

- Apply cold packs to your breasts before and after nursing.

- With your provider's okay, take acetaminophen or ibuprofen.

- Hang in there. If you breastfeed regularly, emptying both breasts every two to three hours, engorgement stops in a day or two. It doesn't take long for your body to match its milk production with your baby's feeding needs.

- If you're not breastfeeding, expect engorgement to last a couple of days until your body gets the message that milk isn't needed. Avoid expressing during this time because doing so just leads to the production of more milk. Applying ice packs and wearing a supportive bra can help with breast discomfort.

RECUPERATING FROM A C-SECTION

The c-section incision in your belly is closed up in several layers after your baby is delivered. The skin layer—the outer layer—is often closed with staples, which are removed right before you leave the hospital. If you have stitches in the skin, they dissolve over time and do not need to be removed. Sutures used in layers beneath the skin are made of material that dissolves, so nothing else needs to be removed.

After surgery, you may feel soreness at the incision site. While you are in the hospital, you may have intravenous medications to control the pain. After three or four days, you will likely go home with oral pain relievers, such as acetaminophen and oxycodone or acetaminophen with codeine. After about a week, ibuprofen or acetaminophen alone can usually relieve the pain.

Your pain should lessen each day. If you start to feel sustained severe pain that gets worse, not better, talk to your provider to see whether the pain is a sign of a problem.

Although soreness is normal at the incision site, excessive pain may mean the cut is becoming infected. This doesn't usually happen, but it's worth knowing about just in case. Signs of infection include pain, chills, and fever, and redness, pus, or swelling around the incision site. If any of these happen, call your provider right away. Infections are more common in women who are obese or who have diabetes. If there is an infection, it can be treated with antibiotics.

Prior to surgery, you had a catheter placed in your bladder to drain your urine. It will probably be left in for the first 12 to 24 hours after surgery so you can relax, rest, and regain feeling in your lower body (if you've had an epidural). Once the catheter is removed, you will need to get up and pee more often—a benefit, since this motivates you to get up and out of bed.

Moving around may be the last thing in the world you feel like doing. But when the nurse or your provider suggests that you get up and go for a short walk around your room or in the hospital hallway, try to do it. There are a few reasons for this.

After a c-section, you have a small chance of developing dangerous blood clots in the pelvis, legs, or chest, especially if you are obese. Moving around speeds up your blood flow and helps prevent clots from forming.

Walking helps your body get rid of gas that built up after the surgery and helps to get your intestinal tract moving. The anesthesia that you were given to block the pain during surgery can make your bowels sluggish, and it's important that they begin to work again. Move around, but don't exert yourself too much.

After a c-section, new mothers usually stay in the hospital for three or four days. Before you leave, ask your provider about activities you should avoid. Driving is usually restricted for about two weeks, and heavy lifting (anything heavier than the baby) and intense exercise should be avoided for four to six weeks. You shouldn't have sex for six weeks either, until after your postpartum checkup. (If you do have sex, use a condom—you can get pregnant in the postpartum period.)

Your body's been through a lot, and it needs nutrients to build itself back up. Be sure to eat right and continue to take your prenatal vitamins after delivery—at least until they run out (when you can switch to regular multivitamins).

WHEN YOU GET HOME

If this is your first baby, you've got to create a whole new set of routines: Where does your baby sleep? Where do you breastfeed? Where do you give your baby a bath? Even if you're an experienced mom, a new baby changes your family. How can you take care of everyone's needs?

As you care for your new baby, remember to care for yourself, too. That means eating, sleeping, and finding time to talk to your partner, your family, and your friends.

Make sure to schedule some you-time, even if it's just a half hour here and an hour there. While your partner or a trusted sitter takes care of your baby, have a coffee date with a friend, go to the movies, take a walk, have your nails done—it doesn't really matter what you do, as long as you have some time to yourself. That downtime can reduce stress and help you feel refreshed and better able to adapt to your responsibilities as a new mother.

Don't expect to be able to do everything on your own. You don't have to be the perfect mom who takes care of her baby, gets herself back in shape, gets dinner on the table, and has a perfectly clean home without any help. Your priority right now is to make sure you and your baby get the best care possible. Ask your partner, family, neighbors, and friends for help and support. Most people love to help, even in small ways. Have a list of specific jobs in mind for helpers—for example, go grocery shopping on Tuesday, make meals to stock the freezer, take the dog for a walk in the afternoon, do a load or two of laundry, take care of the baby for half an hour so you can take a walk. If you find it hard to ask for help, think of it this way: assistance from others frees you up to be a better mother to your baby.

Here are some other ways to care for yourself during the first few weeks after giving birth:

Prioritize sleep Being well rested is essential to your physical and emotional health. Fatigue and exhaustion make it harder for you to care for your baby and yourself. When you're tired, you feel more stressed and less able to handle the challenges of having a newborn. You lack the energy you need to eat well and exercise. You're also more likely to feel depressed, tense, and irritable when you don't get the sleep you need.

As often as possible, follow the old adage, *Sleep when your baby sleeps*. At naptime it's tempting to catch up on household chores that are tough to do while your baby is awake. But if you can possibly manage it, grab a nap when your baby naps. Ask your partner or family members to help with meal preparation, laundry, house cleaning, and other chores so you can get the sleep you need.

Eat well Getting nutritious meals on the table can be a challenge with a new baby. Eating right is vitally important, though—especially if you're breastfeeding. Your body needs nutritious foods—lean protein, whole grains, calcium-rich dairy foods, and vitamin- and mineral-packed fruits and vegetables. (For a review of healthy eating, see chapter 3.)

Simplicity is the secret to smart eating during the busy postpartum weeks. Instead of planning elaborate meals, choose simple, ready-to-eat foods that are naturally nutritious. Some great choices include yogurt, fresh fruit, granola, cold cereal, eggs, low-fat milk, pasta with tomato sauce, vegetable soup, precut salads, cheese and whole-grain crackers, raw vegetables dipped in hummus or guacamole, beans and rice, and peanut butter sandwiches.

Take your time During pregnancy you gained 20 pounds or more. Some of that extra weight is gone now that your baby is born, but new mothers are often surprised at how much weight remains after birth. Some of it is fluid that your body gets rid of on its own. The rest should be lost gradually. If you're breastfeeding and try to lose weight too quickly, it can affect your milk supply. And if you cut back drastically on calories, you risk getting too few of the nutrients you need for breastfeeding, for your own daily needs, and to restock the stores of nutrients that you may have used up during pregnancy.

If you're breastfeeding, you need about 500 calories a day more than you needed before you got pregnant. If you're not breastfeeding, aim for healthy preconception calorie counts. At your six-week postpartum visit, your provider can help you set healthy weight goals.

Typically, women lose about 10 pounds in the hospital and another 10 by their six-week postpartum health-care visit. If you combine healthy eating and moderate exercise, you should be able to return to your preconception weight in a reasonable amount of time.

Move Exercise makes you feel stronger, strengthens and firms up your muscles, strengthens your heart and lungs, helps you feel less tired, energizes you, relieves stress, and helps you return to your preconception weight.

Start taking walks, even if at first you're just walking around the house or yard. Don't feel frustrated if you can't go far or fast. That comes with time. As you feel better, you can do more—but don't overdo it! Listen to your body, and if you feel like you're pushing too hard, slow down.

Consider taking postpartum exercise classes that are offered at hospitals, community centers, and fitness centers. They're a great place to get fit and to meet other mothers of newborns. For a review of smart exercise guidelines, see chapter 5.

Instead of telling yourself, "I have to do everything perfectly," reframe it as, "I'm going to try my best to be a good mother, but I accept that mistakes are a normal part of parenting."

Don't overdo it Your body has been through a lot. You need exercise, but you also need time to rest and heal. Balance movement with relaxation time. Keep an eye on your vaginal bleeding—if it starts to increase after activity, you may be doing too much.

Talk with your provider about your medications If you take medication for diabetes, high blood pressure, an over- or underactive thyroid, or any other medical condition, talk with your provider about how much medication you should be taking. You may need more or less during the first few months after having your baby, or you may need to adjust your medication for breastfeeding.

Continue to take your prenatal multivitamin Your body still needs extra nutrients, especially if you're breastfeeding, so continue to take your prenatal vitamin while you have some tablets left; then switch to a daily multivitamin.

Q: *When can I start having sex again?*

A: *Providers usually recommend holding off until after your six-week postpartum checkup. Six weeks is recommended because that's how long it takes to heal your perineum, vagina, and c-section scar, if you have one. And pregnancy is possible from the start, as well—something that your body isn't yet ready for. If you do have sex prior to six weeks, be sure to use a condom or other birth control method (with your provider's okay) to prevent having another baby right away.*

Reframe unrealistic thoughts Do you expect yourself to be a perfect mother? Do you assume your newborn will be a perfect baby who hardly ever cries and who sleeps through the night at six weeks? Those kinds of perfectionist expectations are bound to leave you disappointed. You're going to have *lots* of imperfect moments as a mother. And babies are famous for doing exactly what their parents don't want them to do—sleeping all day and staying up all night, for example. If you're expecting perfection from yourself or your baby, think about reframing your expectations. Perfectionist thinking about motherhood is an invitation to disappointment and can raise your risk of postpartum depression.

MANAGING POSTPARTUM SYMPTOMS

Your body still has a ways to go before it gets back to normal. During the first few weeks, you may experience some annoying physical symptoms. Most can be managed fairly easily and get better soon.

Here's what you may be feeling:

Sore nipples Your nipples will soon toughen up, but when you start breastfeeding they may feel a little sore. Some soreness is normal, but if breastfeeding hurts, your baby may not be latching on correctly—your baby should take the areola (darker skin around the nipple) into his or her mouth, not just the nipple. Your provider, your baby's provider, or a lactation consultant can help you learn how to guide your baby to latch on correctly.

Sometimes nipple and breast pain are signs of mastitis, an infection of one or both breasts. Bacteria on your skin and in your baby's mouth can cause an infection by entering your breast through cracks in your nipple. Signs of mastitis include redness and feelings of soreness, hotness, swelling, and hardness in your breast, as well as fever and chills. Call your provider if you suspect mastitis, which can be treated with antibiotics.

Although it may hurt, it's good to keep breastfeeding or pumping breast milk while you have mastitis. This helps keep up your milk supply. Don't worry—your baby can't catch the infection from you.

Fatigue Even the easiest deliveries take a huge amount of energy. It's normal to feel exhausted for several weeks—and then the demands of a newborn are enough to tire anyone out! If you feel down and are having trouble concentrating, enjoying yourself, and sleeping, or if you continue to feel exhausted beyond the several-weeks mark, you may be experiencing postpartum depression. (We'll talk more about postpartum depression later in the chapter.) If these symptoms sound familiar, talk to your provider and think about counseling and possibly medication—which can make you feel a lot better.

Mood swings Don't be surprised if your mood is all over the place during the first few days postpartum. Falling hormone levels can leave you feeling joyful one minute and weepy the next. This should get better after a week or so. If it doesn't, call your provider to make sure it's not postpartum depression.

Hemorrhoids The weight of your baby in your belly and the pressure of pushing during birth can both contribute to hemorrhoids, which are painfully swollen veins in and around the anus. To relieve the soreness of hemorrhoids, soak in a warm bath with Epsom salts daily and ask your provider about using over-the-counter hemorrhoid cream, spray, or moistened pads. If passing bowel movements hurts, ask your provider about using an over-the-counter stool softener. Try not to strain while you're passing stool—not only does it hurt, but it can worsen hemorrhoids.

Constipation When you pass your first postpartum bowel movement, constipation may make you feel like you're having another baby. To help move things along, talk with your provider about using an over-the-counter stool softener. (Better yet, ask for one in the hospital right after your baby is born.) Drink plenty of water, eat high-fiber foods, and move around as much as you can safely manage.

Hair loss During pregnancy, hormones caused the growth of extra hair on your head and body. That hair gradually falls out over several months (or up to a year) postpartum.

Swelling If you had swelling of the feet and lower legs during pregnancy, it may not go down until a couple of weeks after birth. Lying on your left side or with your feet up can help reduce swelling.

Stretch marks These dark marks may have appeared on stretched skin on your belly, thighs, breasts, and buttocks during the later months of pregnancy. Stretch marks lighten over time but usually don't disappear completely. Don't bother with stretch mark creams—there's no proof they work.

POSTPARTUM DEPRESSION: MORE THAN JUST THE BLUES

It's normal to feel a bit blue after your baby is born. The sudden change in hormones after birth can lead to a week or so of moodiness that starts a few days after your baby is born. This is often called the baby blues. But 10 to 20 percent of new moms have more than just a mild case of the blues—their moodiness develops into a more serious condition called postpartum depression (PPD).

PPD can happen at any time after childbirth, although it usually starts during the first three months postpartum. It is a medical condition that can happen to any woman after any pregnancy. In fact, it is the most common health problem for new mothers.

Certain factors raise the risk of PPD—for example, major life stresses (such as a job loss or the death of a loved one), relationship problems, financial worries, a history of mood disorders, and medical problems for you or your baby. But you don't have to have any of these in order to get PPD. Sometimes it just happens.

Lack of social support can also raise PPD risk. Many new mothers feel that they must do everything themselves; they feel awkward asking friends and family for help. Don't be embarrassed—you don't have to be a supermom. Ask for help with household chores, cooking, caring for older children, and getting rides to medical appointments. If you're feeling overwhelmed, talk with your partner or other loved ones. It's important to reach out for help if you need it. Be sure to call your provider if blue feelings last more than a few days, or if you have any of the following symptoms:

- Loss of interest in activities you used to enjoy

- Changes in sleep patterns—sleeping too much or too little, feeling tired all the time, or having insomnia

- Changes in eating habits—eating too much or too little, or not wanting to eat foods you used to enjoy

- Trouble concentrating or coping with everyday life

- Unusual weight gain or loss

- Mood swings

- Feelings of anxiety about your baby's well-being, or loss of interest in your baby

- Feelings of nervousness, irritability, sadness, guilt, despair, anger, or helplessness

- Frequent bouts of crying

- Trouble taking care of yourself or your baby

- Panic attacks

- Thoughts or fears of hurting yourself or your baby

- Thoughts about suicide or death

> **Q:** *What is postpartum psychosis?*
>
> **A:** *In rare cases, women with postpartum depression develop a very serious condition called postpartum psychosis. Women with postpartum psychosis may have hallucinations, violent thoughts, and extreme mood swings, and they are at risk of hurting themselves and their babies. New mothers who are experiencing these symptoms shouldn't feel ashamed and should definitely reach out for help. Postpartum psychosis is a medical condition that can be successfully treated. Get help by calling your provider or 911.*

If you feel depressed, tell your provider. PPD is a medical condition and nothing to be ashamed of. PPD can be treated with talk therapy, antidepressant medication, or both. Several kinds of antidepressants are safe even for breastfeeding mothers.

Ignoring PPD won't make it go away. The sooner you get treatment, the sooner you can feel better.

Postpartum Support International provides information about recognizing PPD, along with contact information for local support groups and other resources. Visit their website (www.postpartum.net) or call (800) 944-4773.

YOUR FIRST POSTPARTUM APPOINTMENT

Most providers ask their patients to come in for a postpartum checkup six weeks after they give birth. During this appointment, your provider checks to make sure your body has recuperated from pregnancy and answers any questions you may have about your body, your health, and future pregnancies.

Here's what to expect at your six-week postpartum visit:

- A physical exam, including assessment of your heart rate, blood pressure, temperature, breathing rate, and pain level (if you are still experiencing any pain)

- A postpregnancy exam of your uterus, cervix, vagina, episiotomy site (if you had one), and c-section incision (if you had one) to make sure your body is where it should be in the healing process

- A breast exam
- A weight check: it's best not to lose pregnancy weight too quickly or too slowly—your provider will weigh you and give you advice about setting and meeting postpregnancy weight goals
- A urine test, which checks for excess sugar, excess protein, and infections
- A check-in about any medications you take and any chronic medical conditions you may have
- A blood test if you are at risk for anemia—low blood count—due to heavy bleeding at delivery or postpartum
- A green light to start having sex again, if your body is ready
- A discussion about your next pregnancy, if you plan to have another baby
- A prescription for birth control, if desired
- Answers to any questions you may have

Q: *When will I get my period again?*

A: *Menstruation starts up in about four to eight weeks in women who aren't breastfeeding. If you are breastfeeding, you may not have a period again for several months—some women don't get one until after they wean their babies off the breast. But breastfeeding mothers can ovulate without knowing it, so it's important to use birth control even if you're not having periods. Talk with your provider about what kind of birth control is best for you. Barrier methods such as condoms and diaphragms are safe, although you may have to have your diaphragm refitted. Some kinds of birth control pills (those that use progesterone only) are fine for breastfeeding moms as long as they are careful to take the pills at the same time every day and never miss a pill.*

Q: *How long should I wait to get pregnant with my next baby?*

A: *For most women, it's best to wait at least 18 months after you deliver before getting pregnant again. This gives your body enough time to get ready physically for another pregnancy. Shorter time intervals between pregnancies may increase the risk of premature birth. However, not all women can wait 18 months because of their age or other reasons. Talk with your provider about what's best for you.*

Preconception

Preparing for a Healthy Pregnancy

The best time to start getting pregnancy health care is *before* you get pregnant.

That may sound odd—why get pregnancy care when you haven't even started trying to have a baby? Shouldn't you just wait until you conceive?

The fact is, seeing a health-care provider a few months before you get pregnant for preconception care is a terrific idea.

Whether you're thinking of becoming a mother for the first time or you already have a couple of children, good preconception care boosts your chances of having a successful pregnancy and a strong, healthy baby.

Paying attention to your health before pregnancy gives you the chance to prepare your body for the demands of conceiving, carrying, and giving birth to a baby. It allows you to get as healthy as possible before you get pregnant—to stop using medications that may hurt a developing baby, get control of medical conditions that can complicate pregnancy, and start making lifestyle choices that are best for you and your baby.

Then, when you do get pregnant, your baby has the healthiest possible environment in which to grow.

As soon as you conceive, things happen quickly. Within the first couple of weeks—before you even know you're pregnant—your baby's arms, legs, heart, and spinal cord start developing. By the time you miss your first period, a significant amount of your baby's development has already happened.

With good preconception care, your body is set to start supporting your healthy pregnancy right from the start.

Your partner can get involved in preconception care, too. He can use the months before pregnancy to work on improving his health and changing his unhealthy lifestyle habits. And you can work together to make your home a safe and healthy place for your newborn.

Taking these steps before you get pregnant is a wonderful gift you can give yourself, your partner, and your baby.

THE FIRST STEP

The simplest, most effective thing you can do to prepare for pregnancy is to start taking a daily multivitamin that contains 400 micrograms of folic acid, a B vitamin. Folic acid helps prevent defects of the neural tube, which eventually becomes a baby's brain and spinal cord. Some studies suggest that folic acid may also lower the risk of cleft lip and palate, heart defects, and preterm birth.

Whether you're thinking of becoming a mother for the first time or you already have a couple of children, good preconception care boosts your chances of having a successful pregnancy and a strong, healthy baby.

If all women of childbearing age got the recommended amount of folic acid from the foods they eat or from vitamin supplements before they got pregnant and during the first months of pregnancy, up to 70 percent of neural tube defects could be prevented.

If you're trying to become pregnant, take a daily multivitamin that contains 400 micrograms of folic acid. Since half of all pregnancies are unplanned, women should really be taking multivitamins with folic acid throughout their childbearing years. You can buy them at a drugstore or grocery store—no prescription is needed. Look for the store brand, which is just as effective as the name brand and is often much cheaper.

When you get pregnant, you should switch to a prenatal vitamin with 600 to 800 micrograms of folic acid.

If you've had neural tube–related problems during previous pregnancies, if you are obese, or if you have preexisting medical conditions such as diabetes, epilepsy, or sickle cell anemia, your provider may recommend taking as much as 1,000 to 4,000 micrograms of folic acid each day. However, unless your provider advises otherwise, stick with 400 micrograms daily during preconception.

You get extra folic acid from certain foods you eat: it is often added to bread, cereal, rice, pasta, and tortillas. It's also found naturally—in the form of folate—in foods such as dark leafy greens, citrus fruits, peanuts, lentils, and black beans. Even if you eat nutritious foods, though, it's still important to take a multivitamin with folic acid during the preconception period, to make sure you're getting enough. For more on folic acid and good nutrition, see chapter 3.

A PRECONCEPTION CHECKUP

Pregnancy is a long journey, and before you set out, it's a great idea to make sure your body is ready for the trip. The best way to do that is to see a healthcare provider for a preconception checkup.

You can get a preconception checkup from your family doctor, an internist, a nurse-practitioner, a certified nurse-midwife, or a doctor who specializes in obstetrics and gynecology (known as an OB-GYN).

A preconception checkup includes a physical exam and an internal exam to check the health of your cervix, ovaries, and vagina. Your provider may do a Pap test to look for abnormal cervical cells and to test for STIs such as gonorrhea, chlamydia, and human papillomavirus (HPV). You may also receive a referral for a mammogram, if you're due for one.

Other tests will be done if you need them. A urine test measures levels of sugar, protein, and white blood cells to rule out diabetes, infections, and kidney problems. Blood tests can determine your blood type and uncover problems that could interfere with pregnancy, such as anemia, thyroid disorders, and infections, including STIs such as human immunodeficiency virus (HIV) and syphilis.

If you aren't up to date on your vaccinations, be ready to roll up your sleeve during your preconception checkup. Your provider will let you know if you need vaccines for any of the following:

- Rubella—also called German measles
- Chickenpox—also called varicella
- Tdap—for tetanus, diphtheria, and pertussis (whooping cough)
- HPV—the most common STI in the United States
- Hepatitis B
- Influenza—most often called flu

TALKING ABOUT YOUR HEALTH

During your preconception checkup, your provider will ask you questions about all aspects of your health, including the following:

Your medical history Include details about your current and past health and your family's health. Be sure to tell your provider about illnesses, infections, surgeries, and other medical problems you've had throughout your life.

Your reproductive history Speak honestly with your provider about your sexual history and any previous pregnancies, abortions, miscarriages, or STIs you've had. It's very important for your baby's health that STIs are treated properly before you get pregnant.

Medications Talk with your provider about any prescription drugs, over-the-counter medicines, herbal remedies, skin-cream medications, and supplements you take. Some can cause birth defects and other problems in a developing baby even if you stop taking them as soon as you find out you're pregnant. If any of your medications are unsafe during pregnancy, your provider may switch you to another drug—many medications have safer alternatives. For a list of some of the most commonly used medications that are dangerous during pregnancy, see chapter 1.

Genetics After asking you about your health and your family's health, your provider will talk with you about the risk of possible genetic conditions linked to family history, age, and ethnic background. Your provider may refer you to a genetic counselor or geneticist who can discuss these issues in more detail. In addition, you may be advised to have blood tests (called carrier screening) that can determine whether you are a carrier of certain genetic conditions. For more on genetics and pregnancy, see chapter 9.

Birth control Depending on what kind of birth control you've been using, your provider may suggest that you wait a short time after you stop using it to try to get pregnant. For example, if you use hormone-based birth control (whether as a pill or a patch), your provider may suggest waiting two or three cycles before you try to get pregnant in order to give your body time to return to its natural cycle. No waiting period is recommended if you use condoms, diaphragms, or other barrier methods. When you stop using birth control, keep track of your periods; this can be helpful in figuring out your due date once you get pregnant.

Birth spacing If you have other children, talk with your provider about timing your next pregnancy. For most women, it's best to wait at least 18 months after you give birth before getting pregnant again. This gives your body time to get ready for another pregnancy. A shorter time between pregnancies may increase the risk of preterm birth. But not all women can wait 18 months, because of their age or other reasons. Talk with your provider about what's best for you.

Chronic medical conditions If you have health problems such as high blood pressure, diabetes, lupus, or other chronic conditions, your provider will help you decide how best to manage them during preconception and pregnancy. You may need to see specialists or make changes in the kinds of care your condition requires when you get pregnant. For example, if you have diabetes, it's very important to have your blood sugar in good control before you get pregnant, because high blood sugar at conception and during early pregnancy can interfere with the development of your baby's heart and spine. Fortunately, good sugar control lowers that risk.

MANAGING CHRONIC MEDICAL CONDITIONS FOR A HEALTHY PREGNANCY

Ideally you'd start your pregnancy in 100 percent perfect health. But in reality, you—like many women—may be living with one or more medical conditions that you've had for months, years, or even your entire life. Most chronic medical conditions can make your pregnancy a bit more complicated and may raise some health risks for you or your baby. But in most cases, there are lots of steps you and your provider can take to maximize your chances of having a successful pregnancy. By keeping their conditions in good control and being especially conscientious with prenatal care, most women with medical conditions can manage their pregnancy well and have a healthy baby.

Planning ahead has big benefits for women with medical conditions. Seeing your provider for a checkup *before* you conceive gives you an opportunity to lay the groundwork for a healthy pregnancy. During a preconception visit, your provider can educate you on how your condition will impact your pregnancy (and vice versa); how you can best prepare your body for pregnancy; and how to fine-tune your condition's treatment strategy to make sure it's appropriate for pregnancy.

Most important, your provider can tell you whether the medications you take for your condition are safe for a developing fetus, and whether alternatives exist for drugs that are not recommended during pregnancy.

If you're pregnant already and didn't have a preconception visit, don't beat yourself up. You still have lots of opportunities to make a difference for yourself and your baby—but do try to see your provider as early in your pregnancy as possible. If your medical condition or any of the drugs you take put your baby at risk, you need to know that as early as possible so you and your provider can respond and make adjustments to your treatments and/or medicines. That way you're doing as much as you can to protect yourself and your baby.

Medical conditions raise the risk of some kinds of pregnancy complications and health problems in babies. Knowing the facts about your particular condition can spur you to take the best possible care of yourself and your baby by eating right, taking prenatal vitamins, gaining the recommended amount of weight, going to all of your prenatal health-care appointments, and staying away from cigarette smoke, alcohol, street drugs, pain medications not prescribed by your doctor, and other dangerous substances that can threaten your pregnancy.

It's true that when you have a medical condition during pregnancy, some things are frustratingly out of your control. For example, your condition may raise the chances of having a baby with birth defects. But that makes it all the more important that you do a great job with things that *are* in your control, such as taking prenatal vitamins with folic acid to lower the risk of neural tube defects, and closely following your provider's recommendations regarding the best way to keep your medical condition in check. As with so many situations in pregnancy, you often have more control than you realize.

Each year, hundreds of thousands of women with medical conditions deliver strong, healthy babies after challenging pregnancies. You can push up your odds of being one of those women by making smart choices now and throughout your pregnancy. In the following pages, we'll tell you about steps you can take to have a successful pregnancy even if you have a medical condition.

Acne

Dermatologists have a range of effective drugs to prescribe for acne; however, some of them are *very dangerous* to a developing fetus. For example, isotretinoin (brand name Accutane) has such a high risk of causing birth defects that women of childbearing age are told to take a pregnancy test before starting the drug and to use two forms of birth control while taking it. Studies have found that as many as 35 percent of infants born to women who took isotretinoin during the first trimester had birth defects in the head, face, heart, or central nervous system. The risks of miscarriage and infant death are also high. The U.S. Food and Drug Administration classifies drugs according to their likelihood of causing injury to a fetus. Isotretinoin is listed in category X, the most dangerous.

Certain other acne medications should also be avoided during pregnancy, although they are not as dangerous as isotretinoin. For example, tetracycline can inhibit bone growth and discolor a baby's teeth. Hormonal therapies such as birth control pills, estrogen, flutamide, and spironolactone can cause problems in a baby's genital development.

As for over-the-counter acne treatments, benzoyl peroxide is believed to be safe during pregnancy. Avoid taking oral salicylic acid, however, because it may raise birth defect risk. Salicylic acid applied to the skin seems to be okay, but use it only in small amounts (for example, use sparingly on your face but not in a full-body peel, which would expose you to high levels of it).

The safest way to manage acne during pregnancy is to stick to the basics:

- Wash your face and other acne-prone areas gently twice a day with mild soap and warm water. Don't scrub—that can make acne worse.

- Use oil-free sunscreens and cosmetics and lotions that are noncomedogenic (in other words, that don't clog pores), and avoid alcohol-based cleaning products that strip away your skin's natural moisture.

- Try not to touch the affected area, because bacteria from your hands can cause acne breakouts.

- If you notice that certain foods or situations trigger acne breakouts, try to avoid them.

- When pimples appear, treat them with benzoyl peroxide creams.

- If your acne is serious, talk with your dermatologist and your prenatal-care provider about how best to treat it without putting your baby at risk.

Asthma

It's important to get your asthma under control before conception and keep it under control while you're pregnant, because if you're not getting enough oxygen, neither is your baby—and that's not good for your baby's developing body and brain. Pregnant women with poorly controlled asthma have a higher chance of developing preeclampsia; their babies have an elevated risk of premature birth, low birthweight, poor fetal growth, breathing difficulties, intellectual disability, and cerebral palsy.

However, if your asthma is well controlled, these risks are about the same as they are in the average pregnant woman without asthma.

Asthma symptoms can be controlled during pregnancy with a treatment plan that includes careful avoidance of asthma triggers and the use of inhaled asthma medications such as albuterol, budesonide, and salmeterol, which are considered relatively safe during pregnancy because only small amounts enter the bloodstream.

The effect of pregnancy on asthma symptoms varies: about a third of women say their symptoms improve during pregnancy, about a third say they worsen, and about a third say they stay the same.

If you see an allergist or immunologist regularly, make an appointment early in your pregnancy (or better yet, before you conceive) to find out the best way to manage your symptoms during pregnancy and to see if you need to make changes to your treatment plan or medications. And talk with your provider about whether to use an air purifier at home.

Asthma attacks are often caused by allergens such as pollen, dust, mold, animal fur or dander, cockroach droppings, smoke, air pollution, and freshly cut grass or raked leaves. Pay attention to what sets off your asthma, and avoid it whenever possible. Keep in mind that your triggers may change during pregnancy. If you have exercise-induced asthma, talk with your provider about whether you should curtail your activities.

Asthma probably won't keep you from doing breathing-based relaxation during labor. Asthma attacks typically don't occur during labor or delivery, but you should pack your inhaler just in case.

Cancer

Although pregnancy isn't a viable option for all cancer survivors, many women who have been successfully treated for a variety of cancers do go on to have healthy pregnancies.

If you are a cancer survivor, it's best to consult your oncologist before conception (or as early in pregnancy as possible) to find out if the effects of your cancer or treatment will impact your ability to conceive a baby and safely carry a pregnancy to term. Some kinds of cancer and cancer treatment can reduce fertility or damage the heart or lungs. Radiation near the uterus can restrict the uterus's ability to stretch properly, increasing risk of premature delivery, having a low-birthweight baby, and miscarriage.

Past chemotherapy and radiation generally don't raise the risk of birth defects, provided you wait the recommended time after completing treatment to get pregnant. If you wait as recommended by your oncologist, your baby will have no greater risk of birth defects than a baby born to an average woman who didn't have cancer treatment.

Your oncologist can also help you decide whether you should get your prenatal care from a maternal-fetal medicine specialist who has experience with cancer survivors. This may not be necessary if your cancer had no effect on your reproductive system. No matter whom you see for prenatal care, be sure your provider is fully aware of your cancer history. Your provider may ask you to track down copies of your cancer-care health records, particularly if you were treated for cancer long ago by a different set of providers or in a different hospital.

Before or during your pregnancy, you may want to meet with a genetic counselor to learn about the likelihood of having a genetic condition that contributes to the risk of cancer and passing it to your baby. Many cancers have no known genetic cause, but some do. You may also want to talk with an oncology social worker or other counselor if you're struggling with fear or anxiety related to pregnancy after cancer. During pregnancy, some survivors face fresh fears of having a cancer recurrence that will interfere with their ability to care for their baby, as well as anxiety about the possibility of dying and leaving their baby without a mother. These fears are normal; making peace with them will help you enjoy your pregnancy and look forward to parenthood in a positive way.

There's no evidence that pregnancy causes breast cancer (or any other kind of cancer) to return.

Diabetes

Diabetes can be a challenging condition to deal with, especially during pregnancy. But there are big benefits to careful diabetes management. If you keep your blood sugar in control, you can boost your odds of having an uncomplicated pregnancy and a healthy baby.

Keeping your blood sugar in a healthy target range *before* you conceive (preferably for three to six months) has a big impact on your chances of having a successful pregnancy, because so much of your baby's development occurs during the early weeks of pregnancy, when many women don't even realize they're pregnant.

Maintaining good blood sugar control reduces your risk of miscarriage, premature birth, and preeclampsia, and it lowers your baby's risk of heart and neural tube defects. A woman with out-of-control diabetes is more likely to have a very large baby (10 pounds or more), which can be difficult to deliver vaginally and has a higher risk of birth injuries.

On the positive side, if you do keep blood sugar in control before and during pregnancy, your baby will have no greater risk of birth defects than a baby born to a mother without diabetes.

Managing diabetes during pregnancy poses some challenges because of the changes that go on in your body as your baby grows and develops. For that reason, it's crucial that you work with a team of prenatal-care providers who can support and educate you. If you have an endocrinologist who sees you for diabetes, make a prenatal appointment if possible, and check in with the endocrinologist as soon as you become pregnant. Work with your diabetes-care provider and your prenatal-care provider to determine who will manage your diabetes while you're pregnant.

For your prenatal care, see a maternal-fetal medicine specialist (perinatologist) or an obstetrician who manages high-risk pregnancies and has experience with diabetic patients. Women with diabetes are considered to have high-risk pregnancies, although that doesn't necessarily mean you'll have problems. To protect yourself and your baby, you need specialized care that focuses on the specific needs and risks of a pregnant woman with diabetes.

Talk with your provider about lining up appointments with a diabetes educator and/or a nutritionist who can educate you about the fine points of managing diabetes during pregnancy. And if you have any ongoing diabetes-related health problems, such as heart disease or vision problems, also schedule an appointment with the providers you usually see for those problems.

Here are some other steps you can take to maintain your health, and your baby's, if you have diabetes and become pregnant:

- Work closely with your provider or a nutritionist to design daily meal plans and to set weight gain and exercise goals. It's best for you and your baby if you stay within recommended weight-gain limits. Doing so will help reduce the risk of pregnancy complications.

- Check your blood sugar frequently, and keep track of your results. Talk with your provider about your specific blood sugar targets, based on your individual health profile—they may vary from your preconception targets and may fluctuate during pregnancy.

- Have your hemoglobin A1C checked as often as your provider recommends. This measurement gives a general sense of how well your blood sugar has been controlled over time.

- Keep track of your food and exercise, because they impact your blood sugar levels. You may need to adjust them to keep your blood sugar stable.

- Insulin is safe during pregnancy because it doesn't cross the placenta. If you use insulin, your doses may need to vary while you're pregnant, because of hormones, changes in your body, increased weight, and other factors. Because you may become somewhat resistant to insulin during pregnancy, you may need significantly more over the course of the pregnancy.

- If you take oral diabetes medication, talk to your provider about balancing its risks and benefits. Your provider may switch you to injected insulin instead.

- Talk with your provider about the medications you take to manage diabetes complications. If they are unsafe for pregnant women, alternatives should be considered.

- With your provider's approval, start (or continue) to exercise. Be sure to adjust your insulin accordingly. If you have certain diabetes-related conditions, such as high blood pressure, heart or eye problems, or damage to blood vessels or nerves, your provider may suggest that you limit your exercise.

Gum Disease

If you have gum disease, have it treated before conception or as early in your pregnancy as possible. Your dental-care provider can perform procedures known as scaling or root planing to remove bacterial toxins, plaque, and tartar from deep within your gums and around the roots of your teeth.

While you're pregnant, you can help prevent gum disease from worsening by maintaining good oral hygiene:

- Eat nutritious foods, brush your teeth twice a day, and floss every day to remove plaque from teeth and gums.

- See your dental-care provider regularly, because the hormonal changes of pregnancy can increase your susceptibility to gum disease. Your provider may recommend having your teeth cleaned more frequently than the usually recommended twice a year.

- Make sure you get enough calcium, protein, phosphorous, and vitamins A, C, and D to help your baby's teeth grow strong.

- Pregnant women with gum disease sometimes experience overgrowths of gum between the teeth. These red, occasionally bloody lumps can be surgically removed after your baby is born.

Hemoglobinopathies

Sickle cell anemia and the various thalassemias are a group of conditions that result from genetic changes that affect hemoglobin, the protein in red blood cells that carries oxygen. People of Mediterranean, Southeast Asian, and African ancestry are at increased risk of carrying gene changes associated with a hemoglobinopathy, so they should consider genetic counseling and/or genetic testing to learn their carrier status.

Women with milder forms of thalassemia can usually get pregnant and have healthy pregnancies. Those with more severe forms may be able to have successful pregnancies but require specialized care to make sure their condition is optimally treated. Women with thalassemia should consider having genetic counseling and carrier testing to determine which type of thalassemia they have and implications for their pregnancies.

Women who have sickle cell anemia can have a healthy pregnancy if they get good prenatal care and their provider monitors their disease closely. However, they do have an increased risk of miscarriage, preterm labor, and having a low-birthweight baby. In addition, their disease may flare up during pregnancy, with more frequent episodes of pain. Hydroxyurea, a drug used to treat sickle cell disease, is not recommended during pregnancy because it raises the risk of birth defects.

People who carry the gene change for sickle cell from one parent and the typical hemoglobin gene from the other parent don't have sickle cell disease. They have what's called sickle cell trait and are sickle cell carriers. If both parents have sickle cell trait, their children each have a 1 in 4 chance of having sickle cell disease. Genetic counseling and carrier testing are recommended for people who have an increased risk of being sickle cell carriers.

High Blood Pressure

Having high blood pressure before you get pregnant increases your chances of developing medical problems and complications during pregnancy, such as stroke, organ damage (especially to the kidneys), low birthweight in your baby, the early separation of the placenta from the wall of the uterus (placental abruption), and premature delivery. High blood pressure is associated with increased risk of preeclampsia, a dangerous pregnancy complication. For a discussion of preeclampsia, see chapter 10.

Despite these risks, pregnant women with high blood pressure can have successful and healthy pregnancies—assuming they control their blood pressure before and during pregnancy.

It's best to see a prenatal-care provider before you conceive or as early in your pregnancy as possible. Having high blood pressure means your pregnancy will be considered high-risk, so be sure to see an obstetrician who specializes in high-risk pregnancies.

One of the topics you'll discuss with your provider is whether the blood pressure medications you take are safe during pregnancy. Current recommendations are for pregnant women to avoid angiotensin-converting enzyme (ACE) inhibitors and angiotensin II (AII) receptor antagonists, as well as aldosterone receptor blockers (ARB), because these may cause birth defects, kidney failure, and dangerously high potassium levels in your baby. Don't stop taking these drugs unless told to do so by your provider; but if you are on them and you discover you are pregnant, contact your provider immediately to let your provider know you are pregnant.

If you have hypertension-related conditions such as kidney disease or diabetes, be sure to see your other specialist providers (preferably before you get pregnant) to discuss the best ways to manage those conditions during pregnancy.

Here are some other ways to help protect yourself and your baby:

- Do your best to keep your blood pressure under control before and during pregnancy. If you are overweight or obese, try to lose weight before pregnancy; after you conceive, do your best to gain no more than the recommended amount of pregnancy weight, which is discussed in chapter 6.

- Talk with your provider about your specific blood pressure goals during pregnancy. Your target blood pressure reading may differ during pregnancy, to ensure that your baby gets enough oxygen.

- A woman's blood pressure typically goes up during the third trimester, whether or not she has high blood pressure. Because yours is already high, your provider may wish to see you more frequently during the third trimester, to monitor you more closely. In addition to measuring your blood pressure during these visits, your provider will check your urine for excess protein (a sign that your blood pressure is impacting your kidneys' ability to function well) and may recommend occasional blood tests to check the health of your liver and kidneys, and ultrasounds to verify that your baby is growing properly.

- Your provider may ask you to use a blood pressure cuff to monitor your blood pressure at home. If so, follow your provider's recommendation on how frequently to check your blood pressure, and notify your provider if your blood pressure goes above your recommended limit. Toward the latter part of your pregnancy, your provider may ask you to keep track of how much your baby moves.

- Call your provider right away if you start to experience headaches, visual changes (such as seeing flashing lights), or swelling of the ankles, feet, hands, face, or legs—these are symptoms of preeclampsia.

Kidney Disease

Much is required of your kidneys while you're pregnant. For example, blood flow to the kidneys during pregnancy increases more than 50 percent, especially during the first and second trimesters, requiring them to substantially boost the speed of their waste-filtering processes. They also must work hard to maintain blood pressure and fluid balance as your body undergoes nine months of tremendous change. During pregnancy, your kidneys enlarge slightly in order to perform all the extra work needed of them.

Pregnancy taxes even the healthiest of kidneys, so it's not surprising that women who begin their pregnancy with kidney disease face some special challenges and risks.

Pregnancy can worsen chronic kidney disease and raise the risk of high blood pressure and the conditions that can accompany it, so it's important to get your prenatal care from an obstetrician who specializes in high-risk pregnancies and has experience managing kidney disease.

For women who are on kidney dialysis or who have had a kidney transplant, pregnancy can increase the challenge of maintaining viable kidney function. It is best to talk to your provider before becoming pregnant to understand the serious nature of the medical risks. Many of the drugs used by kidney patients are unsafe during pregnancy. Women with advanced kidney disease face a very high rate of miscarriage.

Women with polycystic kidney disease have a higher likelihood of having a healthy pregnancy than women with other types of kidney disease. Polycystic kidney disease is an inherited disorder in which cysts form in the kidneys, causing them to enlarge and function poorly over the course of many years. Because polycystic kidney disease is a progressive disease, many younger women of childbearing age tend to be healthy enough to have a safe pregnancy. Genetic changes that contribute to polycystic kidney disease have been discovered, so women should speak with a genetic counselor to learn about testing for themselves and to understand the chances for their baby to be affected.

Women with any kind of kidney disease should carefully investigate the risks of pregnancy before conception. If they do choose to get pregnant, they require careful and extensive monitoring in order to help prevent a variety of complications.

Lupus

With careful planning and good medical care, women with lupus can have safe pregnancies and healthy babies: infants born to mothers with lupus are no more likely to have birth defects or intellectual disabilities than babies born to women without lupus. Ideally your lupus should be under control or in remission before you get pregnant. If you conceive during an active lupus flare, you have an elevated risk of miscarriage, stillbirth, preeclampsia, and other serious complications.

Women with lupus have a higher risk of some pregnancy problems, such as premature birth; in fact, about half of pregnancies to women with lupus end early, and about a third of women with lupus have antibodies that can cause blood clots and other problems in the placenta during the second trimester, necessitating early delivery. Lupus also raises a woman's risk of preeclampsia (a sudden increase in blood pressure), excess protein in the urine, or both— any of which may require immediate delivery of the baby to protect the life of the mother and baby.

About 3 percent of babies born to mothers with lupus have a condition called neonatal lupus, which can cause a rash, abnormal blood counts, and a heartbeat abnormality that can be managed with a pacemaker.

If you have lupus, here are some steps you can take to protect yourself and your baby during pregnancy:

- Get your prenatal health care from a maternal-fetal medicine specialist (an OB-GYN who specializes in high-risk pregnancies) who has experience managing lupus.

- Consider planning to deliver your baby in a hospital with a neonatal intensive care nursery that is staffed and equipped to provide critical care to premature babies. (See chapter 1 for more on nursery levels.)

- Call your provider if you suspect you are experiencing a lupus flare while pregnant. Steroids and other lupus medications can be associated with growth impairment and cleft palate and lip in babies, especially when taken in the first trimester. Talk with your provider about medication risks and benefits so your lupus can be managed in the safest way possible for you and your baby.

- It was once thought that all pregnant women with lupus should take small doses of prednisone during and after pregnancy; however, that is now considered unnecessary for most women.

Migraine Headaches

There's no telling how pregnancy will affect migraines, if you're prone to them. Some women find that their migraines worsen during pregnancy; others are happy to discover that their headaches are milder or occur less frequently. Unfortunately, you won't know which of those groups you'll fall into until you're pregnant.

Although migraines can be agonizing, they don't appear to pose any risk to an unborn baby. Drugs such as ergotamine and zolmitriptan don't appear to increase the risk of birth defects, but they are often avoided during pregnancy because they can cause narrowing of blood vessels and can trigger uterine contractions.

To help prevent migraines, keep track of and avoid your triggers. Common migraine triggers include stress, bright lights, allergens, perfumes and other odors, changes in sleep patterns, exercise, loud noises, cigarette smoke, hunger, and certain foods, especially processed or fermented foods, chocolate, dairy foods, pickled or marinated foods, citrus fruits, foods that contain monosodium glutamate (MSG) or nitrates, alcohol (especially red wine), aged cheese, smoked fish, nuts, onions, and artificial sweeteners. Be aware that during pregnancy your triggers may be different than they were before you got pregnant.

To relieve migraine symptoms, try applying heat or cold to your forehead, over your eyes, or on your neck. Other remedies to try include a cold shower, a nap, exercise, and relaxation strategies such as yoga or meditation. Remedies can vary by person and even on a migraine-by-migraine basis.

Call your provider if it's your first migraine, it's accompanied by a fever or blurred vision, it lasts more than a few hours, or you have recurrent migraines.

Phenylketonuria (Maternal PKU)

Phenylketonuria is a genetic disorder that impacts the body's ability to process a protein called phenylalanine, an amino acid that is present in many foods. If newborns who test positive for PKU are fed a special diet that's low in phenylalanine, they can grow up healthy and with normal intelligence. If not, phenylalanine builds up in their blood and can cause brain damage and intellectual disabilities. Newborn screening for PKU began in the 1960s, and since then many women have been able to take advantage of early detection and treatment.

Most people with PKU must continue to follow a PKU eating plan for life. If they eat a normal diet, blood levels of phenylalanine can become very high. Following a PKU eating plan is especially important for mothers during pregnancy and while breastfeeding, and for youngsters during infancy and childhood. Throughout that time the brain is developing and thus is particularly sensitive to the toxic effects of phenylalanine. Some young adults relax their dietary restrictions somewhat, but if a woman with *untreated* PKU and excessive phenylalanine in her blood becomes pregnant, her baby has a high risk of intellectual disabilities, heart defects, behavior problems, small head size, and low birthweight even if the baby does not have PKU.

If you have PKU, you can protect your baby by taking these steps:

- Follow a PKU diet before conception and during pregnancy. It's best to have your PKU in control and your phenylalanine levels down for at least three months before conception, but you can reduce your baby's risk of intellectual disability even if you switch to a PKU diet during the first weeks of pregnancy. Research has found that women whose blood phenylalanine levels were under control before conception, or by eight to ten weeks of pregnancy at the latest, were as likely to have healthy babies as women without PKU.

- Have weekly blood tests during pregnancy to make sure your phenylalanine levels are on target.

- Work with a provider who specializes in PKU before you conceive or as early in your pregnancy as possible to optimize your chances of having a healthy baby.

- See a nutritionist who can help you follow a PKU diet and make sure you're getting all of the nutrients you need during pregnancy, including folic acid and other B vitamins that help protect against neural tube defects.

- Meet with a genetic counselor who can help you determine the likelihood that your baby will have PKU.

- Have an ultrasound at 18 to 20 weeks to check for normal development of your baby's brain and heart.

Seizure Disorder (Epilepsy)

Women with a seizure disorder can have healthy babies. But if you have a seizure disorder, you do face some increased risks. Because of this, it's very important to have a preconception checkup. Your prenatal-care provider should be an obstetrician who is trained to manage high-risk pregnancies and who has experience treating seizure disorders. You should also continue to see your neurologist or whoever provides your seizure care.

Seizures are unpredictable during pregnancy: some women have them more frequently; others have them less often.

Antiseizure drugs are pretty effective at helping to prevent seizures. However, some antiseizure drugs are safer than others during pregnancy, so you may have to switch. In particular, valproic acid increases the risk of neural tube defects: it should be avoided in favor of another antiseizure medication. If you haven't had a seizure in a while, your provider may recommend cutting down to one medication or even suggest a trial of no medication.

Women with a seizure disorder have a higher risk of many adverse pregnancy outcomes, and it's not entirely clear with some of these whether they're due to the underlying seizure disorder or to the medications used to treat it. Potential complications include vaginal bleeding, preeclampsia, placental abruption, stillbirth, and premature birth. Babies of women with seizure disorders have a higher risk of birth defects such as cleft lip or palate, heart defects, and neural tube defects, as well as low birthweight, small head size, bleeding problems, delays in growth and development, intellectual disability, and seizure disorders later in life.

Despite those risks, it's reassuring to know that most women with seizure disorders have healthy babies.

Thrombophilias

The thrombophilias are a group of disorders in which blood clots too easily. Pregnant women should be tested for thrombophilia if they've had a blood clot or a history of certain pregnancy complications, or if they have a family history of blood clots. Blood tests can show whether a woman has a thrombophilia. If a thrombophilia needs to be treated, providers may prescribe blood-thinning drugs that are safe during pregnancy.

A thrombophilia can be inherited or acquired later in life. Genetic counseling can help assess whether you have an inherited thrombophilia and whether genetic testing is appropriate.

Most women with a tendency to develop clotting can have healthy pregnancies. However, they are more likely to develop a deep vein clot (also called deep venous thrombosis, or DVT) or an embolus. An embolus occurs when pieces of clot break off and lodge in the lung (pulmonary embolus) or brain (stroke). Thrombophilias may also contribute to miscarriage, stillbirth, placental abruption, preeclampsia, poor fetal growth, and preterm birth.

Thyroid Disorders

Women with thyroid disorders can have uncomplicated pregnancies and healthy babies if they continue to take their thyroid medication as recommended by their provider. Most thyroid medicines are safe during pregnancy, with the exception of radioactive iodine (which is sometimes prescribed to treat an overactive thyroid).

When thyroid disease is untreated—either because a woman isn't taking her medication or because she doesn't know she has an under- or overactive thyroid—a pregnant woman is at greater risk for high blood pressure and premature delivery. Her baby has a greater likelihood of having developmental problems in the brain and nervous system.

Women without thyroid disease before pregnancy can develop it during pregnancy or after giving birth.

If you have thyroid disease, you can protect yourself and your baby by taking the following steps:

- Talk with your provider about your thyroid condition during your preconception visit and your prenatal visits.

- Take your thyroid medication as recommended by your provider.

- Follow your provider's advice about monitoring your thyroid function with blood tests during your pregnancy to ensure that you are getting the right amount of thyroid medication; dose adjustments are sometimes necessary during pregnancy.

- Contact your provider if you experience any symptoms of hyperthyroidism (including sudden weight loss, increased sensitivity to heat, rapid heartbeat, shaking hands and fingers, difficulty sleeping, and more frequent bowel movements) or hypothyroidism (unexplained weight gain, constipation, increased sensitivity to cold, depression, muscle weakness, dry skin, and hair loss). These symptoms may be signs that your thyroid medication dose needs adjusting.

OTHER WAYS TO PREPARE

There are many other steps you can take to be as healthy as possible before you get pregnant. Some, such as taking a multivitamin with 400 micrograms of folic acid, are pretty simple. Others, such as quitting smoking, may be a bigger challenge. But they're all worthwhile, because they pave the way for a healthier, happier pregnancy.

Preconception is a good time to examine and improve your lifestyle choices—that is, the choices you make every day about things like eating, smoking, drinking alcohol, getting exercise, using recreational drugs, having safe sex, and wearing a seat belt.

Making smart, health-promoting lifestyle choices before and during pregnancy will raise the likelihood that you'll have a successful pregnancy. And building good habits before you get pregnant makes it easier to choose wisely during pregnancy.

Here are some of the best choices you can make for your health and your baby's during the months leading up to conception.

Stop smoking There's no doubt about it: smoking is dangerous for you and your baby. Quitting can be tough, but it's well worth the effort. Women who quit smoking before or during pregnancy cut their chances of a long list of complications, including ectopic pregnancy, vaginal bleeding, placenta problems, and stillbirth. They also lower their baby's odds of being born too early and too small, and of having asthma and learning disabilities in childhood.

Quitting smoking can also make it easier for you to get pregnant. What's more, it can cut your risk of developing cancer, heart disease, and osteoporosis.

Even if *you* don't smoke, the smoke from other people's cigarettes can hurt you and your baby. Now is a good time to reduce your exposure to secondhand smoke as much as possible. Eliminate smoking from your home by making it a smoke-free zone. If your partner smokes, ask him to do so outdoors—or better yet, encourage him to use pregnancy planning as a motivation to quit smoking.

Stop drinking alcohol Once you start trying to get pregnant, stop drinking. Alcohol can cause permanent damage to a baby during the first weeks of development—in other words, even before you know you're pregnant. There is *no* safe amount of alcohol during pregnancy. If you have a problem with alcohol, it's best to get help before you get pregnant. Your provider can refer you to alcohol treatment programs in your area.

Stop using street drugs Cocaine, marijuana, ecstasy, and other street drugs can make getting pregnant more difficult and can cause severe birth defects. It's important to be completely clean before you conceive. Talk with your healthcare provider about how long it will take for drugs to clear out of your system so that you are completely drug-free when you start trying to get pregnant. The same goes for your partner.

Stop using painkillers If you are using opioid painkillers such as codeine, oxycodone, or hydrocodone—*even if they've been prescribed for you by a health-care provider*—you must stop taking them before you get pregnant. Babies born to women who take these medicines just before conception or in early pregnancy have a higher-than-average rate of several serious birth defects. These drugs can cause dependency, so ask your provider for help getting off them.

IN DEPTH

If You Need Help Quitting

See page 243

Help your partner get clean Smoking, drinking alcohol, using street drugs, and being exposed to harmful workplace chemicals such as mercury and lead can make a man less fertile and damage his sperm.

Practice safe sex It's best for you and your baby to start your pregnancy free of any infections, especially those that are sexually transmitted. STIs during pregnancy can raise the risk of miscarriage, preterm birth, stillbirth, and birth defects. To avoid getting an STI, have safe sex with only one person, and be sure he doesn't have an STI and doesn't have any other sex partners.

Get your partner on board Have an honest talk with your partner about supporting you as you improve your health habits, and about the changes he will make. Sure, you're the one who'll be pregnant, but you shouldn't have to be the only one adopting new health habits. Tell him how much it would mean to you if he'd join in on making the choices necessary to have a healthy pregnancy. Getting ready to start or expand your family should be a shared effort.

Do a chemical check at work and at home Exposure to hazardous substances and chemicals can cause birth defects, miscarriage, and other serious health problems. Before you get pregnant, find out if you or your partner is being exposed to dangerous toxins at work. If you're not sure, describe your work environment and any safety equipment you use to your health-care provider. Your provider can tell you what precautions you should take and whether it's safe for you to keep working there during pregnancy. For more on avoiding environmental toxins, see chapter 8.

Avoid fish that's high in mercury Certain kinds of fish contain levels of mercury that are unsafe for pregnant women. During your preconception period it's best not to eat these kinds of fish, because mercury levels can build up in your body and remain high for some time. See the conclusion of chapter 3 for fish-eating guidelines.

Cut back on coffee Large quantities of caffeine may make it harder for you to get pregnant and stay pregnant. *Moderate* caffeine consumption has not been shown to be harmful, however. Recommendations suggest that you limit yourself to 200 milligrams of caffeine per day. That's about the amount in one 12-ounce cup of coffee.

Speak up if you don't feel safe Physical abuse leads to a surprisingly high number of miscarriages and maternal deaths during pregnancy. If you're being abused physically, emotionally, or sexually, ask your provider for help, or contact the National Domestic Violence Hotline: www.thehotline.org or (800) 799-SAFE (7233). If you're not yet pregnant, think hard about whether you really want to have a baby with this person. Abusive partners often turn out to be abusive parents as well.

Take stock of your emotional health This step is especially important if you have a personal or family history of anxiety, depression, prenatal depression, postpartum depression, bipolar disease, or other mental health issues. If you've been feeling unusually sad, angry, irritable, or anxious, ask your health-care provider for a referral to a specialist who may be able to help you using talk therapy and/or medication. And if you're already on an antidepressant or any other psychiatric medication, don't stop taking it without first consulting your provider, because abruptly stopping certain drugs can be unsafe. If your medication is not advised during pregnancy, your provider can probably switch you to a safer one.

Be safe with food Once you start trying to get pregnant, it's important to avoid foods that may contain risky germs. Brush up on the basics of food safety now, so you'll be good to go when you get pregnant. For more on food safety, see chapter 3.

Get moving Exercise improves overall fitness and increases your body's ability to deliver oxygen to your baby. Being active also helps you have a more comfortable pregnancy. Exercising for 30 minutes on all or most days of the week is a good way to help maintain or lose weight, build fitness, and reduce stress. For more on starting an exercise program, see chapter 5.

Take stock of your weight If you are underweight, overweight, or obese, talk with your provider about whether you should try to attain a healthier weight before conceiving.

If you want to lose weight, talk with your provider or consult a nutritionist about a safe way to do it. Follow a nutritious and balanced reduced-calorie diet and increase your exercise. Don't be tempted to starve the pounds off— eating a minimal-calorie diet that's not medically supervised could affect your ability to conceive.

Women who are underweight may benefit from putting on a few pounds before getting pregnant to decrease the risk of having a premature or low-birthweight (under 5½ pounds) baby. For more on healthy weight, see chapter 6.

Look for ways to reduce stress Do what you can to reduce stress in all areas of your life. For stresses that can't be tamed, practice relaxation tools that can help you cope, such as exercise, meditation, and yoga.

See the dentist Have your teeth cleaned and examined, any cavities filled, and any gum infections treated.

Make time for sleep Being well rested gives you the energy you need to exercise, eat right, and make other healthy changes before you get pregnant.

Keep track of your menstrual cycle Noting on your calendar when your menstrual cycle begins and ends each month helps you figure out when conception is most likely to occur. Once you become pregnant, those dates will guide your provider in determining your due date.

MARK YOUR CALENDAR

You've planned and prepared. You're taking vitamins and feeling good about starting the next stage of your life. You're ready to get pregnant!

Most women are fertile—able to get pregnant—about 14 days after the first day of their menstrual period. That's when ovulation occurs: the ovaries release an egg that is ready to be fertilized by a man's sperm. When you're trying to get pregnant, the best time to have sex is a day or two before ovulation or the day of ovulation. The closer sex is to ovulation, the more likely you are to get pregnant.

There are several ways to know when you're ovulating:

- **Temperature.** Use a special type of thermometer called a "basal body temperature thermometer" or a "fertility thermometer" to take your temperature by mouth every day before you get out of bed. Your temperature will rise by up to 1 degree just as you ovulate. Having intercourse as close as possible to this temperature rise improves your chances of getting pregnant.

- **Cervical mucus.** Pay attention to the mucus in your vagina. It gets thinner, more slippery, clearer, and more plentiful just before ovulation.

- **Ovulation prediction kit.** Ovulation prediction kits test urine for a substance called luteinizing hormone (LH). This hormone increases each month during ovulation and causes the ovary to release an egg. The kit will tell you if your LH is increasing. You can purchase ovulation prediction kits at pharmacies.

If you use the temperature or cervical mucus method, begin tracking changes a few months before you want to get pregnant. If you're using an ovulation prediction kit, begin using it about 10 days after the start of your period.

RELAX AND ENJOY

Try not to get too caught up in watching the calendar and counting days. If you're young and not in a hurry, let pregnancy happen when it happens. Enjoy making love without having to worry about birth control. Think of this time as a kind of honeymoon—a time to be in love with your partner in a special, intimate way. Your life changes when you get pregnant, and parenthood has challenges of its own. Savor your time together without putting too much pressure on yourselves to get pregnant immediately.

Once you start trying to conceive, don't worry if it doesn't happen right away. It's normal for it to take a few months.

If you're still not pregnant after six months, talk with your provider. Depending on your medical history and your age, your provider may recommend that you keep trying or that you see a fertility specialist. Typically the specialist route is recommended to women under age 35 who have been trying to get pregnant for at least a year, and women 35 or older who have been trying to conceive for six months.

To find out if you're pregnant, take a home pregnancy test about two weeks after you think you conceived, or have a pregnancy test at your health-care provider's office. If a home test shows that you're pregnant, call your health-care provider and schedule your first prenatal appointment.

As you embark on the amazing journey of pregnancy, be proud of yourself. By making the decision to take charge of your health before and during pregnancy, you've taken a huge step toward a happy, healthy future for yourself and your baby.

In Depth

Some women want or need extra information about pregnancy-related health concerns. Throughout this book, "In Depth" icons have highlighted topics that are explained in detail in the following section. If you have further questions about your health and your baby's health, check with your provider. Or refer to the March of Dimes information-packed websites, marchofdimes.com (in English) or nacersano.org (in Spanish).

Contents

PRENATAL CARE FOR WOMEN WITHOUT HEALTH INSURANCE

It can be scary being pregnant and uninsured. You may be tempted to skip or delay getting prenatal care because you can't afford it. That's not a good idea, because women who don't get good prenatal care are more likely to have health problems during pregnancy, and their babies have a higher risk of preterm birth, low birthweight, and other complications. If you can't afford prenatal care, you have options. Here are some sources of help:

- For a list of health coverage options available in your state, visit finder .healthcare.gov. This site asks you a few key questions and then provides a menu of coverage choices specific to your situation in your state.

- Medicaid, a state/federal program, offers medical assistance for people with low incomes and disabilities. You must be a U.S. national, citizen, or permanent resident alien to qualify; beyond that, each state sets its own eligibility rules. Even if you weren't eligible before you got pregnant, you may be eligible now because you *are* pregnant. Call your state health department to apply, or go to www.medicaid.gov.

- Individual states have various programs that help with medical care for pregnant women. To find out more, call (800) 311-BABY (2229).

- Community clinics and public hospitals sometimes offer free or reduced-rate care.

- Prenatal-care providers sometimes adjust their rates for patients without insurance. Call your provider's business office to ask about discounts.

- For babies and children, the Children's Health Insurance Program (CHIP) provides free or low-cost health coverage. Visit www.insurekidsnow.gov or call (877) KIDS-NOW (543-7669) to find out more. In some states, pregnant women can also get coverage through CHIP programs.

- The Special Supplemental Nutrition Program for Women, Infants, and Children (WIC) provides financial assistance for food and other needs and offers health-care referrals for women and children with a low income, including pregnant women, breastfeeding women, and children up to five years old. Visit www.fns.usda.gov/wic/ to learn more.

- Federal/state collaboration through the Maternal and Child Health Programs helps to provide health-care services for low-income women who are pregnant, and their children under age 22, especially those with special health-care needs. Contact your state health department for more information.

- Indian Health Service provides health-care services for American Indians and Alaskan Natives and their children. Visit www.ihs.gov for more information.

DRUG SAFETY DURING PREGNANCY

To help women and their providers make the best decisions about whether to use various medications during pregnancy, the U.S. Food and Drug Administration categorizes prescription drugs based on their potential to harm a fetus. (Over-the-counter nonprescription drugs are *not* categorized in this way.) Medications are divided into five categories:

- *Category A drugs* are considered safe during pregnancy.

- *Category B, C, and D drugs* are neither clearly safe nor clearly too harmful for use. These categories include drugs for which there is limited information about safety during pregnancy. It is unethical to test potentially unsafe medications on pregnant women, so we don't know a lot about how the drugs that fall into these middle categories affect pregnant women and unborn babies. For category B, C, and D drugs, providers consider whether the benefits of a particular drug outweigh its potential risk in a specific circumstance. For example, if you get a urinary tract infection, it makes sense to take an antibiotic such as amoxicillin, a category B drug, because the potential risk of taking it is smaller than the potential harm to you and your baby if your urinary tract infection goes untreated and spreads to your kidneys.

- *Category X drugs* are considered dangerous to an unborn baby and absolutely should not be taken during pregnancy. These drugs are known to cause birth defects, and an alternative should be used.

IF YOU NEED HELP QUITTING

Smoking It's hard to quit smoking. But trying to quit is well worth the effort. Even if you tried to quit before and failed, take heart: many women find that quitting is easier when they realize how much it will help their baby's chances of being born healthy and full term.

There's lots of support available for pregnant women who want to quit smoking. Start by talking with your provider about programs in your area. You can also get help from these organizations:

- American Lung Association: www.lungusa.org/stop-smoking/ or (800) LUNG-USA (586-4872)

- American Cancer Society: www.cancer.org/healthy/ or (800) 227-2345

- Smokefree.gov: www.smokefree.gov or (877) 44U-QUIT (448-7848)

Alcohol Alcohol can cause permanent damage to a baby during the first weeks of development—even before you know you're pregnant. There is *no* safe amount of alcohol during pregnancy. If you are pregnant and drinking, your provider can refer you to alcohol treatment programs in your area, or you can contact these organizations for help:

- Alcoholics Anonymous: www.aa.org or check your phone directory for the number of your local AA office

- National Institute on Alcohol Abuse and Alcoholism: www.niaaa.nih.gov

- National Institute on Drug Abuse: www.nida.nih.gov

- National Council on Alcoholism and Drug Dependence: www.ncadd.org or (800) NCA-CALL (622-2255)

- Substance Abuse and Mental Health Services Administration (substance abuse treatment facility locator): www.samhsa.gov

- Alcohol and Drug Addiction Resource Center: www.addict-help.com

Street drugs and prescription medicines Cocaine, marijuana, and ecstasy, as well as prescription painkillers, can cause severe birth defects. If you're using narcotic painkillers such as codeine, oxycodone, or hydrocodone—*even* *if they've been prescribed for you by a health-care provider*—it's very important to talk to your provider and make a plan to stop taking them. Babies born to women who take these drugs just before conception or in early pregnancy have a higher-than-average rate of several serious birth defects, including congenital heart defects, spina bifida, and congenital glaucoma.

These drugs can cause dependency, so you may need professional help to get off them. Ask your health-care provider for help, or contact these organizations for information and advice:

- Alcohol and Drug Addiction Resource Center: www.addict-help.com

- National Institute on Drug Abuse: www.nida.nih.gov

- National Council on Alcoholism and Drug Dependence: www.ncadd.org or (800) NCA-CALL (622-2255)

- Substance Abuse and Mental Health Services Administration (substance abuse treatment facility locator): www.samhsa.gov

---

Tips for Quitting

- *Make a list of reasons why you want to quit. Wanting to have a healthy baby is the best reason of all.*

- *Set a quit date. Mark it on your calendar.*

- *Tell your friends and family you're going to quit. Ask them for their support. Ask them not to smoke, drink alcohol, or do drugs around you.*

- *Toss or give away all your cigarettes, alcohol, and drugs. Get them out of your home and car.*

- *Avoid parties, bars, and other places where you might be tempted to smoke, drink, or do drugs.*

NUTRITION REQUIREMENTS FOR PREGNANT TEENS

If you (or your daughter) are a pregnant or breastfeeding teen (age 14 to 18), eating right is even more important for you than for adults. That's because a teen's body is still growing. To get enough nutrients, a pregnant teen should follow the nutrition advice in chapter 3, and also be sure to take a prenatal vitamin every day. However, teens need even more of certain nutrients than women over 18 who are pregnant or breastfeeding. These nutrients include:

Nutrient	Pregnant teens	Breastfeeding teens	Pregnant/breastfeeding women	Good food sources
Calcium	1,300 mg	1,300 mg	1,000 mg	Dairy foods
Magnesium	400 mg	360 mg	350–360 mg (pregnant) 310–320 mg (breastfeeding)	Nuts, bran cereals
Phosphorus	1,250 mg	1,250 mg	700 mg	Meat, poultry, fish, milk, eggs, nuts, legumes
Zinc	12 mg	13 mg	11 mg (pregnant) 12 mg (breastfeeding)	Seafood, meat, legumes

RECOGNIZING AND AVOIDING
SEXUALLY TRANSMITTED INFECTIONS

Some kinds of infections are spread through sexual contact. Known as sexually transmitted infections (STIs), these can cause pregnancy complications, birth defects, and other kinds of health problems for moms and babies. The best way to prevent STIs is to practice safe sex; for existing infections, early treatment is very important for moms and babies.

Infection	Description	Possible symptoms	Prevention tips
Chlamydia	Bacterial infection that can cause preterm birth, eye infections, and breathing problems in baby	Usually none; sometimes vaginal discharge or pain during urination	Practice safe sex
Genital herpes	Infection caused by the herpes simplex viruses; can cause birth defects and health problems in baby	Blisters and cold sores around the mouth, lips, or genitals; also fever, tiredness, aches, pains, vaginal discharge	Avoid sexual contact (including oral-to-genital) with an infected person and contact with an infected person's saliva; condoms don't offer full protection because sores may occur throughout the genital area
Genital warts	Infection caused by viruses from the human papillomavirus (HPV) family; during pregnancy, warts tend to grow and spread more; in rare cases, can spread from mother to baby	Pink, white, or gray cauliflower-like bumps in the genital area	Avoid having sex with a person who has genital warts; condoms don't offer full protection because warts may occur throughout the genital area; if your partner has genital warts, don't have sex until he's been fully treated; vaccine available, but not recommended for pregnant women
Gonorrhea	Bacterial infection that can cause a woman to have pelvic pain, infertility, and infection of the blood and joints; can cause preterm birth, miscarriage, birth defects	Usually none; sometimes vaginal discharge, burning during urination, vaginal bleeding	Avoid having sex with an infected person; use a condom to reduce risk of catching it from a sex partner; treatment early in pregnancy can reduce risks to mother and baby

Infection	Description	Possible symptoms	Prevention tips
Hepatitis B	Viral infection of the liver that can be passed to baby at birth; may cause liver disease in baby	None; or nausea, vomiting, diarrhea, jaundice, dark-colored urine, pale bowel movements	Women at risk of exposure to hepatitis B (e.g., health-care workers) should have a hepatitis B vaccine, which is considered safe during pregnancy; women should also avoid blood/saliva contact, sharing needles, or having sex with an infected person
Hepatitis C	Viral infection that leads to swelling of the liver; may cause liver disease in baby	None; or abdominal pain, itching, jaundice, fatigue, nausea, vomiting	Don't share needles, tooth-brushes, razors, or nail clippers with an infected person; avoid having sex with an infected person; use a condom to reduce risk of catching it from sex partner; if you're a health-care worker, follow routine precautions to avoid exposure to blood
HIV (human immuno-deficiency virus)	Viral infection that causes AIDS (acquired immune deficiency syndrome), which reduces the body's ability to fight off disease; can be passed from mother to baby	Fever, headache, tiredness, enlarged glands in neck and groin	Avoid having unprotected sex with an infected person; avoid contact with infected blood (e.g., sharing needles)
Syphilis	Infection that crosses the placenta into baby's body; can cause birth defects	Sores in the genital area, rashes, fever	Avoid having sex with or sharing needles with an infected person; use a condom to reduce risk of catching it from sex partner; treatment early in pregnancy can reduce risks to mother and baby
Trichomo-niasis	Infection by a parasite; can cause preterm birth	Foul-smelling yellow-green vaginal discharge, genital itching and redness, pain during urination and sex	Avoid having sex with an infected person; use a condom to reduce risk of catching it from sex partner

EXERCISE GUIDELINES FOR PREGNANT ATHLETES

Healthy women athletes can usually continue to exercise during pregnancy. However, you may have to make some adjustments to your training schedule or intensity.

Some of the physical changes of pregnancy affect your body's ability to perform. For example, your body needs more oxygen during pregnancy, so you may feel short of breath sooner than you used to. Your heart rate and blood volume go up in order to meet the oxygen needs of you and your baby. You may sweat more as your body works hard to keep you and your baby cool. As pregnancy progresses, swelling and weight gain may slow you down. In addition, your growing belly and breasts change your center of gravity, making it easier for you to lose your balance and fall.

Your calorie needs change, too. If you exercise intensely, you may need to eat a lot more than usual to get enough calories for both of you. As for intensity, the current recommendation is to use "perceived exertion" as a guide. Your intensity should be sensible and should never exceed preconception levels. In the past, experts said a woman's heart rate should not go over 140 during pregnancy. But because the resting heart rate varies by person, most experts now agree that a pregnant athlete should work with her provider to set her own individual heart rate guidelines.

If you'd like to continue your athletic training during pregnancy, talk with your provider about setting smart goals for exercise intensity and weight gain. If possible, choose a provider who has experience caring for pregnant athletes.

USING BODY MASS INDEX
TO GAUGE YOUR IDEAL WEIGHT GAIN

Your provider will talk with you about the best weight-gain targets for you based on your personal health profile. But generally, the following formula can be used to determine your recommended pregnancy weight gain.

Start by figuring out your preconception body mass index (BMI). BMI is a calculation that takes your height and weight into account to determine whether you are underweight, normal weight, overweight, or obese. Using your height and your weight at the time of conception, find your BMI on the chart below.

BMI	18	19	20	21	22	23	24	25	26	27	28	29	30
Height	Weight (in pounds)												
4'10"	86	91	96	100	105	110	115	119	124	129	134	138	143
4'11"	89	94	99	104	109	114	119	124	128	133	138	143	148
5'	92	97	102	107	112	118	123	128	133	138	143	148	153
5'1"	95	100	106	111	116	122	127	132	137	143	148	153	158
5'2"	98	104	109	115	120	126	131	136	142	147	153	158	164
5'3"	101	107	113	118	124	130	135	141	146	152	158	163	169
5'4"	105	110	116	122	128	134	140	145	151	157	163	169	174
5'5"	108	114	120	126	132	138	144	150	156	162	168	174	180
5'6"	111	118	124	130	136	142	148	155	161	167	173	179	186
5'7"	114	121	127	134	140	146	153	159	166	172	178	185	191
5'8"	118	125	131	138	144	151	158	164	171	177	184	190	197
5'9"	122	128	135	142	149	155	162	169	176	182	189	196	203
5'10"	125	132	139	146	153	160	167	174	181	188	195	202	209
5'11"	129	136	143	150	157	165	172	179	186	193	200	208	215
6'	133	140	147	154	162	169	177	184	191	199	206	213	221

When you know your preconception BMI, you can use the following chart to help determine your weight status and your recommended pregnancy weight gain.

BMI before pregnancy	Preconception weight status	Recommended weight gain during pregnancy
Less than 18.5	Underweight	28 to 40 pounds
18.5 to 24.9	Normal weight	25 to 35 pounds
25 to 29.9	Overweight	15 to 25 pounds
30 or above	Obese	11 to 20 pounds

You may be surprised at what the BMI chart tells you about your weight. You may not think you're underweight, overweight, or obese even though the chart says you are. Don't rush to judgment. Although BMI is a good tool for measuring weight status, it's not perfect, and it doesn't take into account the fact that people have different types of bodies. For example, fit women who are very muscular may have a higher-than-expected BMI even though nobody would consider them overweight. That's because muscle weighs more than fat.

Also, BMI doesn't take the size of your frame or the thickness of your bones into account, which means small-boned women who wouldn't consider themselves underweight may have a BMI that suggests they weigh too little. Don't rely on BMI alone to make decisions about pregnancy weight gain—instead, talk with your provider for a more accurate picture of where you stand on the weight spectrum.

PREGNANCY AFTER WEIGHT-LOSS SURGERY

If you've undergone weight-loss surgery (also known as bariatric surgery), you can have a healthy pregnancy. But because some kinds of weight-loss surgery make it harder for your body to absorb nutrients from food, you may be prone to nutritional deficiencies in protein, iron, vitamin B_{12}, folic acid, vitamin D, and calcium. You may also be limited in the amount and selection of foods you can eat, which might make it hard for you to get the nutrients and calories you and your baby need during pregnancy. These problems can usually be avoided by working carefully with your provider and, if possible, a nutritionist who can help you find ways to get the nutrients you need, through either a carefully planned diet or supplements (or both).

Meet with your bariatric surgeon before you conceive or early in your pregnancy for recommendations on the steps you can take to have the healthiest possible pregnancy. (For example, if you had a gastric-band procedure, you may have the option of having the band adjusted to allow you to eat more during pregnancy.) During your pregnancy, contact your bariatric surgeon if you have abdominal pain.

Women who have weight-loss surgery are advised to wait at least 12 to 18 months after surgery to conceive. Getting pregnant while you are still in the process of postsurgery weight loss can be risky for your baby.

PREGNANCY ADVICE FOR OBESE WOMEN

One-third of American women are obese when they become pregnant. These women face special challenges: their weight increases their risk and their babies' risk of health problems during and after pregnancy. But if you are obese, it doesn't mean you're definitely going to have an unhealthy pregnancy. By making good choices, you can boost your chances of good health for you and your baby.

Start by getting good prenatal care early in your pregnancy (and preconception care, if you haven't yet gotten pregnant). Close monitoring by your provider can help catch health problems such as diabetes and high blood pressure early, when they are easiest to manage. Because of an increased risk of neural tube defects, you should be extra sure to take your folic acid. In addition, your provider may be able to refer you to a nutritionist, who can help you put together a smart eating plan that helps you gain the safest amount of weight.

If your provider approves, begin exercising. Start small, with brief, slow walks. Gradually increase the length, speed, and frequency of your walks. Even modest exercise can help improve your circulation, strengthen your heart, build stamina, and increase feelings of well-being. Recommendations are for women to exercise at least 30 minutes a day, most or all days of the week—but if you can't do that, do what you can, because every little bit helps. If you have the means to do so, think about signing up for a few sessions with a personal trainer who has experience working with obese women. Or join an exercise class for pregnant women at your local Y, community center, gym, or church. (For more on exercise during pregnancy, see chapter 5.)

No matter what you weigh, you have the ability to make things better. You can start making a positive impact on your health and your baby's future by eating nutritious foods, gaining a good amount of weight, exercising, taking the proper supplements, getting high-quality prenatal care, and following all the other advice in this book.

PREGNANCY ADVICE FOR UNDERWEIGHT WOMEN

Like obese women, underweight women face special challenges when they become pregnant. And like obese women, underweight women have the power to make their pregnancy as healthy as possible.

Getting good prenatal care early in your pregnancy is very important. (If you're not pregnant yet, be sure to have a preconception checkup.) If you're underweight, you may be short on important nutrients that are essential for you and your baby—for example, you may not have enough iron in your blood, which can cause anemia.

Your provider can also help you address health issues that may be preventing you from gaining weight. Some women are just naturally slim. But sometimes, being underweight occurs because of excess stress, disordered eating, or untreated depression and anxiety. If that's the case, your provider can refer you to a mental health provider for specialized treatment.

Low body weight can also be caused by smoking, drinking, and substance abuse. If you're struggling with these habits, your provider can assist you in getting the help you need.

Your provider can also refer you to a nutritionist, who can educate you about improving your diet and gaining enough weight while you're pregnant.

If you start pregnancy underweight, be smart about making healthy changes that can help you gain weight. Underweight women have a higher risk of preterm birth and of having a low-birthweight baby.

Remember, no matter how far along you are in your pregnancy, it's never too late to start making changes that can help you and your baby.

LEAD SAFETY RESOURCES

For information about protecting yourself and your family from lead and for lists of certified lead inspectors and removers in your area, contact:

- Environmental Protection Agency's National Lead Information Center: (800) 424-LEAD (424-5323) or www.epa.gov/lead

- Lead Free Kids: www.leadfreekids.org

- Department of Housing and Urban Development's Office of Healthy Homes and Lead Hazard Control: www.hud.gov/lead

- Consumer Product Safety Commission (for information on recalls of lead-containing toys): (800) 638-2772 or www.cpsc.gov

- Environmental Protection Agency Safe Drinking Water Hotline: (800) 426-4791

- Centers for Disease Control (lead information gateway): www.cdc.gov/lead

- NSF International (for consumer information about accessing community-issued Consumer Confidence Reports on drinking water safety and information about water filters, bottled water, and other food- and water-safety issues): www.nsf.org

HEALTH ADVICE FOR MOMS OF MULTIPLES

Giving birth to more than one baby—twins, triplets, or more—has become much more common over the past two decades. These days, more than 3 percent of babies in the United States are born as multiples. Of those, most (95 percent) are twins.

Multiples form in two ways. *Identical* multiples result when one fertilized egg splits and develops into two or more babies. These babies have the same genes and same sex. *Fraternal* multiples result when two or more separate eggs are fertilized by different sperm. When this happens, each baby usually has his or her own placenta. Fraternal multiples do not have identical genes, and they look no more alike than other siblings.

A woman is more likely to have multiples when she is over 30, has a family history of fraternal multiples, is obese or taller than average, and/or is African American. Multiples are also more common among women who get pregnant using assisted reproductive techniques such as in vitro fertilization, in which eggs are fertilized outside the woman's body and implanted into her uterus by a doctor.

Multiple pregnancies are usually discovered during a first-trimester ultrasound. Physical signs of a multiple pregnancy include rapid weight gain during the first trimester, a larger than expected uterus, severe morning sickness, and extreme breast tenderness.

Being pregnant with multiples puts lots of extra demands on a woman's body. But there are many steps moms can take to have the healthiest possible multiple pregnancy. Start by getting good prenatal care. The health needs of a woman who's pregnant with multiples are different from those of a woman who's having just one baby. When a woman is pregnant with multiples, her provider will usually recommend the following:

- *Eating extra food.* Normal-weight mothers of multiples are usually advised to eat 500 extra calories per day (rather than the 300 recommended for singleton pregnancies).

- *Taking iron supplements.* Because mothers of multiples have a higher risk of iron-deficiency anemia, they may be advised to take a multivitamin or iron supplement that contains at least 30 milligrams of iron.

- ***Gaining extra weight.*** Current guidelines suggest that women of normal weight who are expecting twins should gain 37 to 54 pounds; overweight women, 31 to 50 pounds; and obese women, 25 to 42 pounds. Women with triplets may need to gain even more.

Prenatal care is also important, because moms of multiples face a higher risk of some kinds of complications, such as gestational diabetes, high blood pressure, anemia, preterm labor, the need for a c-section, and having a low-birthweight baby.

Providers monitor moms of multiples very carefully, especially after week 20. Because of a higher risk of preterm labor (half of twins are born preterm), a provider may suggest that a mom of multiples cut back on activity and have frequent ultrasounds to check on the babies' growth.

Twins can be delivered vaginally if they're both positioned correctly (head down) and the pregnancy is uncomplicated. Otherwise, multiples are typically delivered by c-section.

Moms can breastfeed multiples successfully. It's a bit more complicated than breastfeeding a single baby, of course, so moms generally benefit from the guidance and advice of an experienced lactation consultant. The La Leche League is also a good resource for moms who breastfeed multiples. To find out more, go to the La Leche website (www.lllusa.org) or call (877) 4-LALECHE (452-5324).

GETTING HELP WHEN YOU'RE DEPRESSED

If you've been feeling unusually sad, angry, irritable, or anxious, ask your health-care provider for a referral to a specialist who may be able to help you using talk therapy and/or medication. If you're already on antidepressants or any other psychiatric medication and want to become pregnant, don't stop taking those medications without first consulting your provider: it can be unsafe for certain drugs to be stopped abruptly. If your medication is not recommended during pregnancy, your provider may be able to switch you to a safer one.

Plenty of resources for depression are available. Ask your health-care provider for help, or contact these organizations for information and advice:

- National Suicide Prevention Lifeline: www.suicidepreventionlifeline.org or (800) 273-TALK (8255)

- National Institute of Mental Health: www.nimh.nih.gov or (866) 615-6464

- National Alliance on Mental Illness: www.nami.org or (800) 950-NAMI (6264)

For more on emotional health during and after pregnancy, see chapters 10 and 15.

GETTING HELP FOR DOMESTIC VIOLENCE AND ABUSE

Abuse, whether emotional or physical, is never okay. Unfortunately, some women are abused by their partners. Women of all races, ethnic groups, and economic levels are abused.

Abuse often gets worse during pregnancy. Almost one in six pregnant women has been abused by a partner. Partners may become abusive (or increase abusiveness) during pregnancy because they feel upset that the pregnancy was unplanned, stressed at the thought of financially supporting a first baby or another baby, or jealous that a woman's attention will shift from the partner to the baby.

Abuse comes in many forms. An abusive partner may cause emotional pain by name-calling or by blaming a woman for something she hasn't done. An abuser may try to control a woman's behavior by not allowing her to see her family and friends or by always telling her what she should be doing. Emotional abuse may lead a woman to feel scared or depressed, eat an unhealthy diet, or pick up bad habits such as smoking or drinking.

An abusive partner may try to hurt a woman's body. This physical abuse can include hitting, slapping, kicking, choking, pushing, and hair-pulling. Sometimes an abuser will aim these blows at a pregnant woman's belly. This kind of violence can not only harm the mother, but also put the unborn baby in grave danger. During pregnancy, physical abuse can lead to miscarriage and vaginal bleeding. It can cause a baby to be born too soon, have low birthweight, or sustain physical injuries.

If you are hurt by your partner or anyone else, get medical help for yourself and your baby. But you don't have to wait until physical violence happens to get help: if you're worried that your partner may try to hurt you, ask your provider to refer you to a local shelter and to services for victims of domestic violence.

You can also get help from the following:

- National Domestic Violence Hotline: www.thehotline.org or (800) 799-SAFE (7233)

- National Coalition Against Domestic Violence: www.ncadv.org

VAGINAL BIRTH AFTER C-SECTION (VBAC)

Medical experts used to believe that once you had a baby by c-section, all of your future babies would have to be born by c-section. But many medical experts now believe that a vaginal birth after a c-section (VBAC) can be safe for many women and their babies, though there may be some risks. In fact, 70 percent of women who attempt VBAC successfully deliver vaginally.

Some of the benefits of having a VBAC include avoiding surgery, a shorter recovery time, and a lower risk of infection, blood loss, and other c-section health complications.

VBAC is a good choice for many women, but not all. You and your provider can decide if VBAC is right for you. Not all providers and hospitals offer VBACs, so if you're interested in having one, be sure your provider and hospital are on board. In general, you may be able to have a VBAC if:

- You had at least one vaginal birth before or after your last c-section.

- You had a past c-section for a reason that isn't a problem in this pregnancy. For example, you had an infection in your last pregnancy, but not in this pregnancy.

- Your past c-section incision (cut) was made side to side in the lower part of your uterus. (This is called a low transverse incision.)

- You and your baby are in good health during pregnancy.

- Your labor starts on its own, before or on the day that your baby is due.

VBAC can have some risks. These risks include:

- If your labor doesn't go well, you may have to have a c-section anyway.

- Your baby may have a hard time handling the stress of labor.

- If you need to have an emergency (unplanned) c-section after labor starts, you're at increased risk of getting an infection in your uterus.

- Your uterus may tear or even rupture during labor where your past c-section incision was made. This complication is rare, but it can be life-threatening. To make uterine tear or rupture less likely, your health-care provider needs to check your medical history to learn what kind of incision you had in your past c-section and monitor your labor carefully.

LESS COMMON PREGNANCY COMPLICATIONS

Many common complications of pregnancy are discussed in chapter 10. Some of the less common complications are described in the following pages. They occur in only a small number of pregnancies, but it's good to know a few things about them just in case.

Hyperemesis Gravidarum

Morning sickness is a common problem in pregnancy. It's normal to have some nausea and vomiting, especially in early pregnancy. But in rare cases, women develop severe morning sickness that prevents them and their babies from getting the nutrients and water they need. This is called hyperemesis gravidarum (HG), and if you have it, you should take it seriously.

Risk factors. Pregnancy with more than one baby or the presence of an abnormal growth in the uterus called a hydatidiform mole (which results in what's called a molar pregnancy). Though the cause of HG is often unknown, acute morning sickness is believed to be a reaction to the hormones of pregnancy. HG is more common in first-time mothers.

Risks to mom and baby. Lower-than-recommended weight gain (mother); small size and low birthweight (baby).

Symptoms. Severe nausea, vomiting, lightheadedness, loss of appetite, weight loss, dehydration.

Diagnosis. Your provider checks your blood pressure, which is often low in women with HG, and your pulse, which may be high, and does a blood test to determine if you are dehydrated (not getting the water you and your baby need).

Treatment. Your provider may check you into the hospital so that you can receive intravenous fluids and antinausea medication. HG usually starts to improve after the first trimester, although some women have it throughout their pregnancy. Some women find that vitamin B_6 supplements or ginger helps reduce nausea.

Amniotic Fluid Disorders

Amniotic fluid is the clear, watery liquid that surrounds your baby in the amniotic sac. Amniotic fluid passes in and out of your baby's body through breathing, swallowing, and urinating. The fluid helps your baby's lungs and digestive system grow and develop in a healthy way.

Amniotic fluid protects your baby, acting as a cushion and helping to maintain a steady temperature. It also gives your baby a means to move around while inside you, which helps with the development of muscles and bones.

As your baby grows, the amount of amniotic fluid increases. At 36 weeks of pregnancy, you have about one quart of amniotic fluid. As you get closer to giving birth, the amount of fluid begins to decrease.

In some women, the amount of amniotic fluid is too much or too little. Both of these conditions can pose risks for babies.

Polyhydramnios This condition, in which a woman has too much amniotic fluid, can occur if birth defects or other problems prevent the baby from breathing in and swallowing enough fluid. If this condition occurs late in pregnancy, it may not be a problem. But if amniotic fluid starts building up early in the pregnancy, it increases the risk of premature birth.

Risk factors. Birth defects or infection in the baby, poorly controlled diabetes in the mother, or Rh incompatibility. Sometimes polyhydramnios has no known cause, though it is more likely to occur in women carrying more than one baby.

Risks to mom and baby. Early rupture of the amniotic sac, premature birth, placenta problems, poor positioning of the baby for birth, and bleeding after delivery.

Symptoms. Swelling (edema) in the lower extremities from the pressure of the enlarged uterus, and shortness of breath when the amniotic sac enlarges within the uterus, crowding your lungs. Mild polyhydramnios usually has no symptoms.

Diagnosis. Your provider can use an ultrasound to find out whether you have the right amount of amniotic fluid.

Treatment. To lower your amniotic fluid level, your provider can remove some amniotic fluid with a needle or give you a drug that helps reduce it.

Ways to lower your risk. If you have uncontrolled diabetes, keeping your blood sugar at your recommended level can reduce your chance of developing polyhydramnios.

Oligohydramnios The condition in which a woman has too little amniotic fluid, called oligohydramnios, can start at any time, although usually it occurs toward the end of pregnancy or after the due date.

Risk factors. Tears in the amniotic sac, placenta problems, an overdue pregnancy, birth defects in the baby, and conditions such as high blood pressure, diabetes, or lupus.

Risks to mom and baby. If early in pregnancy, birth defects of the lungs and limbs, miscarriage, premature birth, and stillbirth; if in the third trimester, slow growth of the baby, birth complications, and an increased risk of c-section; if near or after the due date, usually no problems.

Symptoms. Small-seeming belly.

Diagnosis. Your provider can use an ultrasound to find out whether you have the right amount of amniotic fluid.

Treatment. Your provider will probably put you on bedrest and watch your baby closely using ultrasounds, nonstress tests, and biophysical profiles. (For more on these tests, see chapter 10.) If the tests suggest problems or the fluid gets too low, delivery will be recommended, either by inducing labor (via medications that cause labor to start) or by c-section. In some cases, a provider can replace fluid by putting a plastic tube into the uterus and infusing fluids. This is called amnioinfusion. This treatment works only to protect the baby during labor, however, because the fluids leak right out.

Ways to lower your risk. Drink plenty of water. If you have health conditions such as high blood pressure or diabetes, do your best to manage them.

Placenta Disorders

The placenta is a pancake-shaped, blood-filled organ that grows inside your uterus. One side of the placenta is attached to your uterus and connects to your blood supply. The other side connects to your baby by the umbilical cord. The placenta, which looks like a blood-filled sponge, serves as your baby's life-support system. It supplies your baby with nutrients and oxygen from your blood. It also moves waste from your baby's blood to your blood, where it is then eliminated by the kidneys.

Early in pregnancy, the placenta is usually low in the uterus. As your baby grows, the placenta usually moves up; and by the time birth occurs, it is high in the uterus. After birth you no longer need the placenta, so it is expelled by your body shortly after your baby is born.

Sometimes the placenta can develop problems that are dangerous to you and your baby. Most placental problems involve serious bleeding.

Placenta previa In the condition known as placenta previa, the placenta is so low in the uterus that it covers all or part of the internal opening of the cervix, blocking the opening through which a baby must pass during birth. When the placenta blocks the cervix, having a vaginal birth becomes difficult or dangerous, because severe bleeding can occur as the cervix starts to open if the placenta detaches from the uterus (placental abruption).

Risk factors. Smoking or using street drugs, being over age 35, having an abnormally developed uterus or placenta, being pregnant with more than one baby, having had several previous pregnancies, and scarring in the uterus caused by previous surgeries or births.

Risks to mom and baby. Placental abruption (see below), which may involve heavy vaginal bleeding that requires delivery (and that reduces blood supply for both mom and baby), premature birth, stillbirth, and complications during birth.

Symptoms. Sudden heavy vaginal bleeding (painless or with cramps) beginning in the later weeks of the second trimester, or no symptoms at all.

Diagnosis. Your provider can do an ultrasound to check on the position of your placenta.

Treatment. If you have placenta previa, the condition may correct itself as your uterus grows and pulls the placenta up away from the cervix. If it doesn't, your provider may recommend hospitalization during the last weeks of pregnancy. Birth by c-section can protect you and your baby by preventing excessive blood loss.

Ways to lower your risk. Don't smoke or use street drugs. Be sure to tell your provider if you've had uterine surgery of any kind.

Placental abruption This is a very serious condition in which the placenta separates from the wall of the uterus, partly or completely, before birth. If your placenta separates from your uterus, your baby may not get enough oxygen and nutrients. Because of the heightened chance of excessive bleeding, placental abruption can be life-threatening to you and your baby.

Risk factors. High blood pressure, habits such as smoking and using street drugs (particularly cocaine), injury to the belly (for example, in a car accident or domestic violence), age over 35, pregnancy with more than one baby, infection in the uterus, abnormality of the uterus (such as fibroids), abnormality of the placenta, abnormality of the umbilical cord, early rupture of membranes (having your water break early), polyhydramnios, a prior placental abruption, certain blood-clotting disorders, and having a very small baby.

Risks to mom and baby. Premature birth, stillbirth, complications during birth, and intellectual disabilities in the baby.

Symptoms. Sudden constant pain and cramping in the abdomen and sudden bleeding. Sometimes there is no bleeding because the placenta is blocking the cervix and thus prevents blood from flowing out of your body.

Diagnosis. Your provider can use an ultrasound to check for placental abruption.

Treatment. If the abruption is mild, your provider may recommend bedrest, either at home or in the hospital. If it is more serious, your provider may advise early delivery, either by inducing labor (giving medications that cause labor to start) or often by c-section, especially if there is a lot of blood loss.

Ways to lower your risk. If you have high blood pressure, do your best to keep it under control. Stay away from cigarettes and street drugs, wear a seat belt to protect yourself in the event of a car accident, and seek help and protection if you are at risk for domestic violence.

Placenta accreta, placenta increta, and placenta percreta These are conditions in which the placenta attaches itself so deeply and firmly into the wall of your uterus that it does not separate easily from your uterus after you give birth.

Risk factors. Having scarring in the uterus from a previous c-section or uterine surgery; having placenta previa in the current pregnancy.

Risks to mom and baby. Premature birth and excessive bleeding in the mother, as well as miscarriage, poor growth of the baby, premature birth, and birth defects.

Symptoms. Vaginal bleeding, usually in the third trimester.

Diagnosis. Your provider can look for these placenta disorders using an ultrasound or magnetic resonance imaging (MRI). MRI is a noninvasive test that uses magnetic power and radio waves to produce images of organs and structures inside your body. MRI is considered safe to use during pregnancy (better than CT—computed tomography—scans) as a way to diagnose potentially dangerous health conditions.

Treatment. Your provider may recommend early delivery by c-section; after vaginal birth, surgical removal of the placenta is often needed. In some cases, a hysterectomy (surgical removal of the uterus) is necessary to prevent dangerous blood loss.

Ways to lower your risk. Although these conditions are fairly rare, they have become more common as the c-section rate has gone up over the past few decades, because having a previous c-section is a risk factor. Having a c-section only when it is medically needed can protect you from unnecessary risks in later pregnancies.

Umbilical Cord Abnormalities

The umbilical cord is a narrow tube that connects a baby to the placenta. Blood vessels in the umbilical cord work as a transportation system between mother and baby. Blood, nutrients, and oxygen flow from the placenta to the baby through the umbilical cord; the baby's waste products flow out through the umbilical cord to the placenta, where they are carried away by the mother's blood. The umbilical cord reaches a length of about 22 to 24 inches by about 28 weeks of pregnancy.

Problems with the umbilical cord can cause problems for mother and baby during pregnancy or birth. Potential problems include the following:

- *A cord that's too long.* A long cord can wrap around the baby's limbs or neck (the latter causing a condition called nuchal cord). Cord wrapping happens normally in 25 percent of babies and rarely causes problems. A long cord may also get knotted; this too is usually not a problem, although in some cases—if the knot gets too tight and prevents blood from flowing to the baby—delivery by c-section is required.

- *A cord that's too short.* A short cord may prevent the baby from being delivered vaginally if it won't let the baby move far enough down the birth canal.

- *A cord that's improperly connected.* If the umbilical cord doesn't connect well to the placenta, it may tear during labor and delivery, leading to heavy bleeding (and overall blood loss for the baby and mother).

- *A cord containing a single umbilical artery.* The umbilical cord usually contains three blood vessels: one vein and two arteries. Sometimes a cord develops with only two blood vessels: one vein and only one artery. (This occurs more often when a woman is pregnant with more than one baby.) If the single umbilical artery is an isolated finding, the baby is usually fine. If it is associated with other findings on ultrasound, such as birth defects in the heart, nervous system, and urinary tract, an amniocentesis should be considered to look for an underlying genetic cause.

Deep Vein Thrombosis

Deep vein thrombosis (DVT) is a condition in which a blood clot forms in one of the veins deep within a lower leg or thigh. The clot, called a thrombus when it stays where it formed, can block blood flow in the leg, causing pain and swelling. If it (or a piece of it) breaks away and travels through the bloodstream, it's called an embolus. If a traveling clot reaches a major organ and blocks circulation there, it can cause serious damage or even death: for example, a clot can cause a pulmonary embolism (PE) in the lungs, a stroke in the brain, or a heart attack in the heart. Blood clots in the lungs are the number one cause of death in pregnant women in the United States.

Risk factors. DVT is more likely to occur in people with a family history of DVT or of blood-clotting disorders known as thrombophilias, because their bodies make either too much of the proteins that help blood clot or not enough of the proteins that stop blood from clotting. DVT can also occur in people who sit or lie still for long periods of time, which allows blood to pool in the legs. Being pregnant raises DVT risk because of natural changes in blood that occur during pregnancy and increase its tendency to clot; that risk remains higher than normal until about six weeks after birth.

Risks to mom and baby. Organ damage to the mother, and death to mother and baby.

Symptoms. Swelling, pain, and tenderness in the leg (or wherever the DVT is located); skin that is warm to the touch, red, or discolored. If the clot travels to a lung, symptoms include shortness of breath, pain with breathing, and rapid heartbeat.

Diagnosis. An ultrasound can show whether blood is flowing normally, and blood tests can tell whether your blood contains a substance that's produced by blood clots. X-rays and blood tests may also be used.

Treatment. Medications can thin the blood and dissolve blood clots. If you have a DVT lodged in a leg, a vein filter may be implanted between the leg and your heart to stop the blood clot (or parts of it) from traveling to the heart, lungs, or other organs.

Ways to lower your risk. Avoid sitting or lying in one position for long periods of time. On car, train, and plane trips lasting more than four hours, stand up and walk around every hour or so. While sitting, occasionally flex and stretch your feet to increase blood flow in your calves, a common site of DVT. Compression stockings can also help stop blood from clotting in the legs. Drink plenty of water, gain the recommended amount of pregnancy weight, and don't smoke. If you're on bedrest, ask your provider what activities you can safely do to boost blood flow in your legs without putting your baby at risk.

Liver Disorders

The liver is an organ located in your upper-right abdomen. Your liver cleans up your blood and helps you digest and use food. To help do its work, your liver produces fluid called bile, which your body needs to absorb the fats in the foods you eat. When your liver doesn't work correctly during pregnancy, it can cause problems for you and your baby.

Acute fatty liver This is a rare condition in which fat builds up in the liver of a pregnant mother.

Risk factors. Genetic problems that prevent the body from processing fat properly.

Risks to mom and baby. Coma, organ failure, and death in mother and baby. Babies born to mothers with this disorder must be fed a special low-fat diet to prevent the development of life-threatening problems in the liver, heart, and muscles. In the mother, the disorder usually goes away within a few days after birth.

Symptoms. Persistent nausea and vomiting, pain in the stomach or upper-right abdomen, fatigue, yellowing of the skin and the whites of the eyes, and headache.

Diagnosis. Your provider can identify this condition with blood tests that look at liver and kidney function.

Treatment. Mothers with acute fatty liver may require transfusions until the baby can be delivered.

Ways to lower your risk. There are no known ways to prevent this condition.

Intrahepatic cholestasis of pregnancy (ICP) This is a condition in which high levels of bile acid build up in the mother's blood. This can cause severe itching of the skin, usually during the second or third trimester.

Risk factors. ICP in a previous pregnancy, pregnancy with more than one baby, and a family history of liver disorders.

Risks to mom and baby. Itching so acute that it disrupts sleep or work, jaundice (due to excess bilirubin, which is related to bile), premature birth, and stillbirth.

Symptoms. Itchy skin on the palms of your hands, the soles of your feet, and other parts of your body; yellowing of the skin and the whites of your eyes (a sign of jaundice).

Diagnosis. Your provider uses a simple blood test to check how well your liver is working several times during pregnancy (and more often if you have symptoms).

Treatment. Your provider can prescribe a medication that helps your liver work better, relieves itching, and may help prevent stillbirth. The condition usually disappears after delivery, although it may come back in future pregnancies.

Ways to lower your risk. There are no known ways to prevent ICP.

Molar Pregnancy

A molar pregnancy is created when mistakes occur as a sperm and an egg meet for fertilization.

There are two kinds of molar pregnancy: complete and partial. When a molar pregnancy is complete, there is no embryo. When a molar pregnancy is partial, the uterus contains abnormal placental tissue and an abnormal embryo. A molar pregnancy may be followed by a more serious condition called gestational trophoblastic disease.

Risk factors. Being an adolescent, being white, being over age 40, and having had previous miscarriages or molar pregnancies.

Risks to mom and baby. Even if there is an embryo present along with the abnormal placental tissue—in other words, a partial molar pregnancy—that embryo will not develop into a baby. Women who have had a molar pregnancy frequently go on to have normal pregnancies and healthy babies in the future.

Symptoms. Severe nausea and vomiting (morning sickness or hyperemesis gravidarum), dark-colored vaginal bleeding or spotting early in pregnancy, loose stools, rapid heartbeat, shaking hands, unexplained weight loss, nervousness, high blood pressure, and swelling in the ankles, feet, and legs.

Diagnosis. Your provider can use an ultrasound and other types of scans to look for an abnormal mass, along with a blood test to measure hormone levels (which can be abnormal during a molar pregnancy) and to check for problems with the kidneys, liver, and blood clotting.

Treatment. Your provider can use one of two procedures—a dilation and curettage (D&C) or a suction curettage—to remove the mass from your uterus. After removing the mass, your provider will send it to a laboratory to be checked for cancerous cells, which are present in 20 percent of these cases.

If the mole has spread extensively, your provider may suggest a hysterectomy, a surgical procedure in which the entire uterus is removed.

Women who have a molar pregnancy should not get pregnant again for six months to one year. During that time, your provider will use blood tests to make sure that pregnancy hormone levels have returned to normal and that the mole hasn't started growing again. If there is evidence of growth, medication called methotrexate can be given to stop it.

Ectopic Pregnancy

After a man's sperm fertilizes a woman's egg, the early embryo is supposed to travel to the woman's uterus and plant itself on the inside wall of the uterus. Sometimes the fertilized egg implants in the fallopian tubes instead (or, rarely, the ovaries, cervix, abdominal cavity, or outside surface of the uterus). This is called an ectopic pregnancy.

Risk factors. A history of sexually transmitted infections such as chlamydia (which can cause scarring in the fallopian tubes and thus slow down the embryo as it moves from ovary to uterus), previous ectopic pregnancy, fertility treatments, damage to the fallopian tubes because of surgery or tubal sterilization, endometriosis (a condition in which uterine tissue grows beyond the uterus), exposure to tobacco smoke, and a woman's exposure to the drug DES (diethylstilbestrol, a synthetic estrogen) when *her* mother was pregnant.

Risks to mom and baby. It is impossible for a baby to develop outside the uterus, so ectopic pregnancies can't result in the birth of a baby. They can also endanger the mother's life by causing internal bleeding. Many women who have ectopic pregnancies go on to have normal pregnancies and healthy babies in the future, although they do have a higher-than-average risk of another ectopic pregnancy.

Symptoms. Irregular brownish vaginal bleeding about a week after a missed period, with pain on one side of the lower belly followed by severe pelvic pain, shoulder pain, faintness, dizziness, nausea, or vomiting. An ectopic pregnancy can be dangerous, so it's important to call your provider or go to the hospital if you have these symptoms.

Diagnosis. Your provider will use a pelvic exam, blood tests to measure pregnancy hormones (which are often low during an ectopic pregnancy), and an ultrasound to locate the pregnancy.

Treatment. The pregnancy must be surgically removed before it causes a rupture of the fallopian tube and excessive bleeding that can threaten the mother's life. (If ectopic pregnancy is diagnosed early enough in the pregnancy, medication can be used instead of surgery to stop the early pregnancy from growing and rupturing the fallopian tube.)

Glossary

Pregnancy Words to Know

afterbirth: The placenta that comes out of the vagina after a vaginal birth. The placenta grows in your uterus and supplies food and oxygen to your baby through the umbilical cord during pregnancy.

afterbirth pain: Belly cramps caused when your uterus goes back to its regular size after pregnancy.

amnio: See *amniocentesis.*

amniocentesis: Also called an amnio. A test that takes some amniotic fluid from around your baby in the uterus. The test checks for problems with the baby, such as birth defects or genetic problems. You can get this test at 15 to 20 weeks of pregnancy.

amniotic fluid: The fluid that surrounds the baby in your uterus.

amniotic sac: The sac (bag) inside the uterus that holds a growing baby. It is filled with amniotic fluid.

anemia: When the body doesn't have enough red blood cells or the red blood cells are too small. Women get anemia when they don't have enough iron in their bodies. Anemia is common in pregnancy.

antepartum: Before birth.

antibiotic: A medicine that kills infections caused by bacteria.

antibodies: Cells in the body that fight off infections.

anus: The opening through which bowel movements leave the body.

Apgar test: A test done on your baby right after birth. The test checks five things to make sure your baby is healthy: heart rate, breathing, muscle tone, reflexes, and skin color.

areola: The dark area around the nipple on each breast. It may get darker or larger during pregnancy.

baby blues: Feelings of sadness in the first week or two after having a baby.

bacteria: Tiny organisms that live in and around your body. Some bacteria are good for your body, and others can make you sick.

bedrest: A significant reduction in activity while you're pregnant. Bedrest may mean staying in bed all day or just resting a few times each day.

bikini cut: A cut used in surgery that goes horizontally across your belly, just above your pubic bone. It may be used in c-sections.

birth canal: See *vagina*.

birth control: Also called contraception or family planning. Things you can do, such as using a condom or taking birth control pills, to keep from getting pregnant.

birth defects: Problems with a baby's body that are present at birth.

bladder: Where your body holds urine.

bleeding: Also called spotting. When blood comes out of your vagina during pregnancy.

blood test: A test of your blood to check for sugar, infections, and other possible problems.

blood transfusion: The process of getting new blood in your body via an intravenous line.

bloody show: Bleeding from your vagina at the beginning of labor.

BMI: See *body mass index*.

body mass index: Also called BMI. A measure of body fat based on your height and weight. It can help you find out if you need to gain or lose weight.

bowel movement: Solid waste that leaves the body through the anus.

Braxton Hicks contractions: Also called false labor. Contractions that help prepare your body for labor. They are different from labor contractions in that they don't get stronger or happen faster over time and they may stop when you move around.

breastfeeding: Feeding your baby milk that comes from your breasts.

breast milk: Milk that comes from your breasts. Breast milk is the best food for a baby.

breast pump: A pump used to help remove breast milk from your breasts to feed your baby via a bottle.

breech position: When the baby's bottom or feet (rather than head) are facing down right before birth.

catheter: A tube used to drain urine from your bladder.

cerclage: A stitch that your doctor puts in your cervix to help keep it closed so that the baby isn't born too early.

certified nurse-midwife: Also called a CNM. A nurse who has special education and training to care for pregnant women and deliver babies.

cervix: The opening to the uterus that sits at the top of the vagina.

cesarean birth: Also called a c-section. Surgery in which your baby is born through a cut that your doctor makes in your belly and uterus.

CF: See *cystic fibrosis.*

childbirth classes: Classes for you and your partner to learn about what happens during the birth of a baby.

chloasma: Also called the mask of pregnancy, or melasma. When the skin around a woman's eyes, nose, or cheeks turns brown or gets darker during pregnancy. It usually goes away after pregnancy.

chorionic villus sampling: Also called CVS. A test of tissue from the placenta that checks for birth defects and genetic problems, such as Down syndrome. You can get CVS at 10 to 13 weeks of pregnancy.

chronic health condition: A health condition that lasts for a long time or that happens again and again over a long period of time. Examples are diabetes, high blood pressure, obesity, and depression.

circumcision: Removing the foreskin from the penis.

CMV: See *cytomegalovirus.*

CNM: See *certified nurse-midwife.*

colostrum: A sticky, yellowish fluid that comes out of your breasts right after you give birth, before your breast milk comes in. It feeds your baby and helps protect your baby from infection. Your body starts making colostrum during the last few months of pregnancy.

conception: Also called fertilization. When a man's sperm gets inside a woman's egg. This is how a woman gets pregnant.

constipation: When it's hard to have a bowel movement.

contraception: See *birth control.*

contraction: When the muscles of your uterus get tight and then relax. Contractions help push your baby out of your uterus.

cord blood: Also called umbilical cord blood. The blood remaining in the umbilical cord and placenta after the baby is born and the cord is cut.

crib death: See *sudden infant death syndrome.*

c-section: See *cesarean birth.*

CVS: See *chorionic villus sampling.*

cystic fibrosis: Also called CF. A disease that affects breathing and digestion. Parents with a CF gene change can pass the disease to their children.

cytomegalovirus: Also called CMV. A virus that is a common cause of infection in young children. Most of the time it does not cause problems. But if a pregnant woman gets infected, she can pass it to her baby. If this happens, the baby could get very sick, have lifelong problems, or even die.

D&C: See *dilation and curettage.*

dehydration: Not having enough water in your body.

depression: A medical condition in which strong feelings of sadness last for long periods of time and prevent a person from leading a normal life.

diabetes: Having too much sugar in your blood. Excess blood sugar can damage organs in your body, including blood vessels, nerves, eyes, and kidneys.

diagnostic test: A medical test that tells you if you do or do not have a certain health condition. It's different from a screening test, which tells you if you're more likely than other people to have a certain health condition.

dilate: To open up. Your cervix dilates to let the baby out.

dilation and curettage: Also called a D&C. When a doctor removes tissue from the lining of a woman's uterus. Some women have a D&C after a miscarriage.

domestic violence: When your partner abuses or hurts you. It can be emotional abuse, as when your partner yells at you or calls you names. It also can be physical abuse, like hitting, kicking, or punching.

Doppler fetal monitor: Also known as a Doppler. A kind of ultrasound device that can measure a baby's heart rate by detecting blood flow.

doula: A person who has special training to help you handle labor.

Down syndrome: A genetic disorder that includes a combination of birth defects, such as intellectual disability, heart defects, certain facial features, and hearing and vision problems.

due date: The estimated date that you will have your baby. It is about 40 weeks from the first day of your last period.

ectopic pregnancy: When a fertilized egg implants itself outside of the uterus and begins to grow. An ectopic pregnancy cannot result in the birth of a baby. It can cause dangerous problems for the pregnant woman. Most of the time, ectopic pregnancies are removed by surgery.

edema: Swelling. Many pregnant women have swelling in the legs, feet, ankles, hands, and face.

efface: To thin out. Your cervix effaces to let the baby out.

egg: Also called an ovum. During ovulation, a woman's ovaries release an egg. When a woman's egg is fertilized by a man's sperm, the woman gets pregnant.

ejaculation: When semen—liquid containing millions of sperm—comes out of a man's penis.

embryo: A fertilized egg that results when an egg and a sperm combine. The embryo implants itself into the wall of the uterus and grows to become a fetus.

engorgement: When your breasts become full of milk.

epidural: Pain medicine you get through a thin tube in your lower back that helps numb your lower body during labor. It is the most common kind of pain relief used during labor.

episiotomy: A cut made at the opening of the vagina to help let the baby out.

fallopian tubes: The tubes between your ovaries and your uterus. When an ovary releases an egg, it travels down one of these tubes to your uterus.

false labor: See *Braxton Hicks contractions.*

false negative: A test result (from a blood test, for example) that tells you a problem does not exist when in reality it does.

false positive: A test result (from a blood test, for example) that tells you a problem exists when in reality it does not.

family history: A list of questions a health-care provider asks to find out about diseases and other health problems in your family, and your responses to those questions.

family planning: See *birth control.*

FASD: See *fetal alcohol spectrum disorders.*

fertility specialist: Also called a reproductive endocrinologist. A medical doctor who is an expert in helping women get pregnant.

fertilization: See *conception.*

fetal alcohol spectrum disorders: Also called FASD. When a baby is born with physical and mental birth defects caused when the mother drinks alcohol during pregnancy.

fetal fibronectin test: Also called an fFN test. A test you may get to see if you are in preterm labor. It checks to see how much fFN protein you have in your vagina. If the test shows that you don't have any fFN, you probably won't have your baby for at least another two weeks.

fetal monitor: A device placed on your belly during labor to check contractions and the baby's heartbeat.

fetus: A growing baby from eight weeks of pregnancy until birth.

fFN test: See *fetal fibronectin test.*

first-trimester screening: Tests to see if your baby is more likely than other babies to have certain birth defects, including heart problems and Down syndrome. It's usually done at 11 to 13 weeks of pregnancy. It includes a blood test and an ultrasound.

folic acid: A vitamin, sometimes called folate, that can help protect your baby from neural tube defects.

forceps: A tool that can be used to help deliver a baby. Forceps look like big tongs.

formula: A milk product that you can feed your baby instead of breast milk.

full term: A pregnancy that lasts between 37 and 42 weeks. It's best for your baby if you stay pregnant until your baby is full term.

gene: A part of each cell in your body that stores instructions for the way your body grows and works. Genes are passed from parents to children.

genetic: Having to do with things that run in families, like eye or hair color or certain diseases.

genetic counselor: A person who is trained to know about genetics, birth defects, and medical problems that run in families.

genetic disorder: A condition caused by a gene that has changed from its regular form. A person's gene can change on its own, or a changed gene can be passed from parents to children.

genetic test: A medical test that looks for changes in genes that can cause birth defects or other medical problems.

gestational age: The number of weeks a baby has been in the uterus.

gestational diabetes: A form of diabetes that some women get during pregnancy.

glucose screening test: A test to see if you have diabetes.

group B strep test: A prenatal test for group B strep, a bacterial infection of the vagina that can hurt your baby.

hCG: See *human chorionic gonadotropin.*

health-care provider: Also called a provider. The person who gives you medical care. Your provider could be a doctor, a nurse, a certified nurse-midwife, a nurse-practitioner, or another trained medical professional.

health insurance: Helps you pay for medical care. You may get health insurance from where you work, get it from the government, or buy it on your own.

heartburn: A burning feeling in your chest caused by stomach acid.

hemorrhoids: Swollen veins in and around the anus that may hurt or bleed. Hemorrhoids are common during and after pregnancy.

hepatitis B: A disease caused by a virus that attacks the liver. Pregnant women get tested to see if they have it. Most babies get a vaccination before they leave the hospital so they won't get the disease.

herb: A plant used in cooking and medicine. Examples of herbs used as medicine are mint, chamomile, and ginkgo biloba. Do not use herbs as medicine during pregnancy.

high blood pressure: Also called hypertension. When the force of blood against the walls of the blood vessels is too high. High blood pressure can cause problems during pregnancy.

high-risk pregnancy: A pregnancy that is more likely than other pregnancies to have problems. Things that can make a pregnancy high-risk for a woman include having a medical problem like diabetes or high blood pressure and being over- or underweight.

hormones: Chemicals made by one part of the body that send a signal to another part of the body.

human chorionic gonadotropin: Also called hCG. A hormone that a woman's body makes during pregnancy.

hypertension: See *high blood pressure.*

immune: Being protected from a specific infection. If you're immune to an infection, it means you can't get that infection.

implantation: When a fertilized egg (embryo) attaches to the lining of the uterus and begins to grow.

incision: A cut made by a surgeon or other doctor. For example, a surgeon makes an incision in your belly and uterus through which to deliver your baby by a c-section.

incompetent cervix: When the cervix opens too early, before the baby is full term.

incontinence: Not being able to control when you urinate.

induce labor: When your provider gives you medicine and/or breaks your amniotic sac to help your body start labor.

infection: An illness you get from some viruses and bacteria. Some common infections are the flu, chickenpox, HIV, and vaginal infections. Infections can cause problems during pregnancy.

infertility: Not being able to get pregnant.

intravenous: Also called an IV. When medicine is given through a needle into a vein. During labor, many women have an IV put into their arm so they can get liquids and medicine directly.

IV: See *intravenous.*

jaundice: When a baby's eyes and skin look yellow. A baby has jaundice when his liver isn't fully developed or isn't working well.

Kegel: An exercise that strengthens pelvic muscles. It can help prepare the muscles for labor and delivery.

lactate: To produce milk in the breasts. A lactating mother is able to breast-feed her baby.

lactation: See *breastfeeding.*

lactation consultant: Someone who has special training in helping women breastfeed.

limb buds: The parts of a developing baby that become the arms and legs.

linea nigra: A dark line on the belly that some women get during pregnancy. It goes from the belly button down to the pubic area.

lochia: See *vaginal discharge.*

mask of pregnancy: See *chloasma.*

maternal blood screening: A test of your blood to see if your baby is more likely than other babies to have some birth defects.

maternity/maternal: Having to do with being pregnant or being a mother.

meconium: A baby's first bowel movement. It can be green, brown, or black in color.

Medicaid: A government program that pays for medical care for people with very low incomes.

melasma: See *chloasma*.

membrane: Tissue that connects the amniotic sac to the uterus.

menstrual cycle: The recurring monthly process in which an egg is produced by an ovary and moves through the fallopian tube to the uterus. If the egg is not fertilized by sperm, it passes through the vagina along with blood from the uterus. This discharge is called a period.

menstruation: Also called a period. The bleeding you have at the end of your menstrual cycle. If you get your period each month, you're not pregnant.

mercury: A metal that is often found in oceans, lakes, and rivers. You can get mercury in your body by eating certain kinds of fish.

metabolism: How well and fast your body processes what you eat and drink.

mineral: An inorganic substance, such as iron and calcium, that helps your body work and stay healthy. You get minerals from foods or from a vitamin pill.

miscarriage: When a baby dies in the uterus before 20 weeks of pregnancy.

morning sickness: Feeling sick to your stomach during the first few months of pregnancy. Even though it is called morning sickness, it can last all day.

mucus: A thick fluid that coats and protects parts of the body.

mucus plug: A mass of mucus that blocks the opening of the cervix. It helps keep the baby safe from infection.

multiples: More than one baby in the same pregnancy.

multivitamin: A pill that contains many vitamins (such as vitamins B and C) and minerals (such as iron and calcium) that help the body work and stay healthy.

narcotic: An opioid drug that relieves pain.

nausea: Upset stomach.

neonatal intensive care unit: Also called a NICU. A section of a hospital that takes care of sick newborns.

neonate: A newborn baby up to four weeks old.

neural tube: The part of a developing baby that becomes the brain and spinal cord.

newborn screening: Blood and hearing tests your baby has before leaving the hospital to check for certain treatable problems that may occur during childhood.

nicotine: A drug that is found in cigarettes. Nicotine can be harmful to a developing baby.

NICU: See *neonatal intensive care unit.*

NP: See *nurse-practitioner.*

nuchal translucency: The fluid at the back of an unborn baby's neck. An ultrasound can measure the thickness of this fluid to help find out if the baby has certain birth defects, such as Down syndrome.

nurse-practitioner: Also called an NP. A registered nurse with advanced medical education and training.

nutrients: Components of food that help your body work and stay healthy.

obesity: Extreme overweight.

OB-GYN: See *obstetrician-gynecologist.*

obstetrician-gynecologist: Also called an OB-GYN. A doctor who has special training to care for women, including pregnant women.

operating room: A room in a hospital where surgery is done.

ovaries: Where eggs are stored in the female body. Women have two ovaries, one on each side of the uterus.

over-the-counter medicine: Medicines, such as aspirin or cough syrup, that you can buy without a prescription.

ovulate: To release an egg into a fallopian tube.

ovum: See *egg.*

Pap smear: Also called a Pap test. A medical test in which a provider collects cells from a woman's cervix. The cells are looked at under a microscope to check for signs of cancer.

Pap test: See *Pap smear.*

pasteurized: In the case of food or drink, having been heated to kill bad germs. Milk and juice usually are pasteurized.

paternity/paternal: Having to do with a baby's biological father.

pediatrician: A doctor who has special training in taking care of babies and children.

pelvic area: The part of the body between the stomach and the legs.

pelvic exam: An exam of the pelvic organs to make sure they are healthy.

pelvic organs: Organs in the pelvic area, including (for women) the vagina, cervix, uterus, fallopian tubes, ovaries, and bladder.

pelvic pressure: The feeling that your baby is pushing down inside you. Pelvic pressure is a sign of preterm labor.

penis: A man's primary sex organ.

perinatal: The period of time before and after a baby is born, from the 20th week of gestation to the 28th day after birth.

perineum: The area between the vagina and the rectum/anus.

period: See *menstruation.*

placenta: An organ that grows in your uterus and supplies the baby with food and oxygen through the umbilical cord.

postpartum: Having to do with the time after a baby's birth.

postpartum depression: A medical condition in which a woman has strong feelings of sadness that last for an extended period of time after her baby is born.

preconception: The time before pregnancy.

preconception checkup: A medical checkup to help make sure you are healthy before you get pregnant.

preeclampsia: A certain kind of high blood pressure that only pregnant women get.

premature baby: A baby born before 37 completed weeks of pregnancy.

premature birth: Birth that happens too early, before 37 completed weeks of pregnancy.

prenatal care: Medical care you get during pregnancy.

prenatal tests: Tests that you and your baby get during pregnancy. They help your provider find out how you and your baby are doing.

prenatal vitamin: A vitamin made especially for pregnant women, with dosages targeted at mother/baby health.

prescription: An order for medicine written by a health-care provider.

preterm labor: Labor that happens too early, before 37 completed weeks of pregnancy.

progesterone: A hormone that, when given to a pregnant woman, can help prevent preterm labor. The type of progesterone used for this purpose is called 17P.

provider: See *health-care provider.*

quickening: The time during pregnancy when you can begin to feel your baby move. It usually happens in the second trimester of pregnancy.

rectum: Where bowel movements are stored before they leave the body.

reproductive endocrinologist: See *fertility specialist.*

Rh disease: A disease of newborns caused when a baby who is Rh-positive is born to a mother who is Rh-negative and who has not received Rh treatment. See *Rh factor.*

Rh factor: A protein found on red blood cells. If you have the protein, you are Rh-positive. If you don't have it, you are Rh-negative. Most people are Rh-positive. If a woman is Rh-negative and her baby is Rh-positive, her baby may be born with a disease called Rh disease. A woman can be tested and treated during pregnancy to make sure her baby isn't born with Rh disease.

risk factor: A known reason why something could go wrong. For example, smoking is a risk factor for having a premature baby. If you smoke, you're more likely than women who don't smoke to have a premature baby.

safe sex: Using a condom if you have sex with more than one partner, or with an infected partner, to help make sure you don't get a sexually transmitted infection such as HIV or herpes.

screening: A medical test, often a blood test, to see if you are more likely than other people to have a certain health condition. It is different from a diagnostic test, which tells you if you do or do not have a certain health condition.

secondhand smoke: Smoke you breathe in from someone else's cigarette, cigar, or pipe.

sexually transmitted infection: Also called an STI. An infection you can get from having sex with someone who has the infection. Examples of STIs are chlamydia, gonorrhea, syphilis, HIV, and herpes.

side effect: An effect of a drug or medicine that is not the *intended* result. For example, a side effect of some cold medicines is that they make you sleepy.

SIDS: See *sudden infant death syndrome.*

speculum: A tool that a health-care provider uses to hold the vagina open during a pelvic exam.

sperm: During ejaculation, a man releases sperm. When a woman's egg is fertilized by a man's sperm, the woman gets pregnant.

spinal block: A shot you can get in your lower back that numbs your lower body. Many women choose to have a spinal block during labor and delivery.

spotting: See *bleeding.*

STI: See *sexually transmitted infection.*

stillbirth: When a baby dies in the uterus before birth, but after 20 weeks of pregnancy.

stretch marks: Lines you get on your skin when it stretches. During pregnancy, you may get stretch marks on your belly, thighs, breasts, and bottom.

sudden infant death syndrome: Also called SIDS. The unexplained sudden death of a baby.

supplement: Something you take in addition to what you eat that helps your body work and stay healthy. Examples include vitamins (such as vitamins B and C) and minerals (such as iron and calcium).

support group: A group of people who have the same kinds of concerns. They meet together to try to help one another.

teratogen: A drug or chemical a pregnant woman takes or is exposed to that can cause her baby to have a birth defect.

thyroid: A gland in the neck that makes hormones that affect your heart rate, your metabolism, and other aspects of your health.

toxoplasmosis: An infection you can get from eating undercooked meat or touching infected cat feces.

transverse position: When the baby's shoulder is facing down right before birth.

trimester: A time period of about three months. Pregnancy is divided into three trimesters: first, second, and third trimesters.

ultrasound: A device that uses sound waves and a computer screen to make a picture of a baby in the uterus. Also, an assessment of the baby that employs such a device.

umbilical cord: The cord that connects the baby to the placenta. It carries food and oxygen from the placenta to the baby.

umbilical cord blood: See *cord blood.*

umbilical cord prolapse: When the umbilical cord slips into the vagina, where it could be squeezed or flattened during vaginal delivery.

urinary problem: A sensation of pain or burning when you urinate, or the inability to urinate.

urination: When urine leaves the body.

uterus: Also called a womb. The place inside you where your baby grows.

vaccination: A shot that contains a vaccine.

vaccine: Medicine you or your baby gets that protects against certain diseases.

vagina: Also called a birth canal. The baby comes out of your vagina during a vaginal birth.

vaginal birth: The way most babies are born. During vaginal birth, the uterus contracts to help push the baby out through the vagina.

vaginal birth after cesarean: Also called a VBAC. When you have a vaginal birth after having had a cesarean birth in an earlier pregnancy.

vaginal discharge: Mucus that comes out of your vagina. Vaginal discharge may increase during and after pregnancy.

varicose veins: Swollen veins.

VBAC: See *vaginal birth after cesarean.*

virus: A tiny organism that can make you sick. Viruses cause diseases such as measles, colds, the flu, and AIDS.

vitamin: A nutrient that helps the body work and stay healthy. You get vitamins such as vitamin A, vitamin C, and many others from the foods you eat and/or from vitamin pills you take.

WIC: Stands for Women, Infants, and Children. WIC is a program run by the U.S. government that helps provide financial assistance for food and other needs for women and children with a low income, including pregnant women, breastfeeding women, and children up to five years old.

womb: See *uterus.*

Index

blood tests, 14, 82, 137
  prenatal, 13–15, 125
  for newborns, 180
blood volume increase, 25, 35, 94
"bloody show," 137
bloody stool, 86
body aches, 87, 88, 91, 94
body mass index (BMI), 70
  calculating, 70
  gauging your ideal weight and, 249–50
BRAT diet, 39
Braxton Hicks contractions (false labor), 163
breastfeeding, 153, 187–94
  advantages, 187–88
  birth control use during, 192
  birth control pills and, 211
  infant stools and, 196
  learning how, 188–89
  medication use during, 191
  for moms of multiples, 256
  nutrition and calorie needs, 191, 204
  positions for, 192
  Q&A, 189–94
  resources for, 193
  sore nipples, 206
breasts. *See also* breastfeeding
  changes in, 93–94
  engorgement, 201
  leakage of colostrum, 31, 94
  month-by-month, 24, 25, 30, 31
  postpartum, 197, 200–201
  tips to relieve discomfort, 94
  when to call your provider, 94, 208
breathing difficulty, 31, 95
  shortness of breath, 137
  when to call your provider, 91, 95, 208
breech position, 166
  c-section and, 166
  external cephalic version and, 166

caffeine, 46, 85
  cutting back on coffee, 235
calcium, 35, 38, 104, 251
  dairy foods and, 43
  foods high in, 35, 38, 78
  for pregnant teens, 245
  supplements, 35
  vegetarianism and, 43
cancer, getting pregnant and, 221–22
carrier screening, 119, 121–24
car safety seat, 156–57
certified nurse-midwives (CNMs), 8

cervical insufficiency (incompetent cervix), 138
cervix
  labor and, 166, 170, 171, 172
  month 9 of pregnancy, 32
cesarean birth (c-section), 174–76
  breech position and, 166
  by choice, 176
  medical reasons for, 174–75
  percentage of U.S. births, 162, 176
  recuperating from, 201–2
  risks, 174
  vaginal birth after (VBAC), 176, 259
  what to expect during, 175
childbirth, 161–77
  assisted delivery, 172
  back labor, 168
  birth plan for, 155–56
  breech position and, 166
  crowning, 172
  by c-section, 162, 163, 174–76
  delivery and birth, 172–73
  delivery injuries, 172, 176, 222
  doula for, 154
  epidural for, 169, 171
  episiotomy, 172, 173
  exercise to help, 65
  fetal monitoring, 169–70, 171
  getting ready, 162–63
  high-risk baby, 132
  hospital nursery classification, 20
  labor, 163–64, 170–73
  labor, induced, 165–67
  medication for pain (chart), 169
  nesting, 165
  next pregnancy following, 211
  obesity and c-section, 69–70
  pain, coping with, 167–69, 171
  pain medication and, 162, 169
  passing urine, gas, or stool during, 171
  postpartum symptoms, managing, 206–7
  recovering from, 197–211
  relaxation techniques, 167–68, 171
  rupture of membranes, 164–65
  umbilical cord, 172
  vaginal birth, 163–73
  when to go to the hospital, 164, 171
  where to have your baby, 19–21
childbirth classes, 152–53
Children's Health Insurance Program (CHIP), 156, 240
chloasma or the mask of pregnancy, 92

exercise *(continued)*
  for mood swings, 96
  postpartum, 204–5
  preconception, 235
  prenatal fitness classes, 63
  prenatal yoga, 64
  preterm birth risk, lowering and, 62
  sit-ups while pregnant, 68
  sleep affected by, 82
  strategies to make it fun, 61
  tips for safety, 66–68
  turning a walk into a workout, 61–63
  walking, calories burned, 77
  when to stop exercising, 67
  who should not exercise, 61

faintness, 87, 91, 105, 137, 208, 269
family physicians, 7
fatigue, 24, 25, 26, 79, 80
  anemia and, 82, 137
  gestational diabetes and, 139
  postpartum, 206–7
fetal alcohol spectrum disorders (FASDs), 17
fetal development
  absence of, or decreased movement, 67,
    91, 149, 177
  brain growth, third trimester, 44
  kick count, 177
  month-by-month, 24–32
  movement, 27, 28, 30, 31, 32, 176–77
fetal growth restriction, 70
fetal heart defects, 131, 132, 222
fetal monitoring, 169–70, 171, 177
fish. *See* seafood
flu (influenza), 57
  flu shot, 15, 57, 216
folic acid (folate), 11, 35, 38, 214, 251
  foods high in, 35, 38, 41, 78, 215
  fortification of grain and cereal, 3–4
  supplements, 3, 11, 35, 214–15
food allergies, 47–48
food-borne infections, 49–54
  E. coli, 52
  foods to avoid, 49, 50–51, 52
  listeriosis, 50–51
  meat thermometer to protect against, 53
  prevention, 55
  salmonellosis, 51–52
  toxoplasmosis, 53–54
  washing to prevent, 52
food cravings/preferences, 24, 47
formula feeding, 194–96

fragile X syndrome, 124
full-term pregnancy, length, 8

gas (flatulence), 79, 84, 85
genes and human genetics, 120–21
  autosomal dominant inheritance,
    122–23
  sex chromosome abnormalities, 130
  single gene disorders, 130
  X-linked inheritance, 124
genetic screening, 13
gestational diabetes (GD), 19, 69, 139–40
gestational throphoblastic disease, 268
glucose, 36
gum disease, 224, 236

hair
  growth of, in odd places, 79, 93
  loss, postpartum, 207
  safe removal methods, 93
headaches, 26, 89–90, 141
  migraines, 89, 90, 228–29
  over-the-counter pain relievers, 90
  when to call your provider, 90, 91, 98
health insurance, 9, 72, 158
  adding your baby to policy, 156
health proxy, 159
heart beat or rate (baby's), 18
  bradycardia, 170
  contraction stress test, 177
  falling, c-section and, 174
  fetal monitoring, 169–70, 171, 177
  hearing for first time, 26
  nonstress test, 177
  normal, 170
heartburn, 27, 46, 79, 80, 84
  medication, 85
  relieving, 39, 84–85
hemoglobinopathies, 224
hemophilia, 124
hemorrhoids, 80, 83, 85–86, 207
hepatitis B, 14
  vaccination, 216
herbal products, 13, 48
high blood pressure (chronic), 6
  getting pregnant with, 225–26
  medications, safety of, 225
  when to call your provider, 226
high blood pressure (pregnancy-related), 19,
    61, 140–42
high-risk pregnancies
  frequency of prenatal appointments, 18

hospital birth for, 19–20
NICUs and, 20, 132, 180
providers for, 7, 8, 13
what it is, 19
HIV/AIDS, 14, 19, 247
home births, 21
hormones
avoiding products with, 12
blood volume increase and, 94
breathing and, 95
discomforts of pregnancy and, 79, 80, 82, 83
emotions and, 95
migraines and, 89
mother's, month 1 of pregnancy, 24
sweating, postpartum, and, 199
hospital birth, 19–20
classification of nurseries, 20
NICUs, 20, 132, 180
planning for high-risk baby, 132
hyperemesis gravidarum (HG), 87, 260

infections
bacterial vaginosis, 56
common cold, 56
complications and, 15, 55, 138
cytomegalo-virus, 56
flu, 15, 57, 216
parvovirus B19 (fifth disease), 57
postpartum, 200, 202
prevention, 55–59
rubella (German measles), 14–15, 57
strep, A or B, 57
TB, 58
UTI, 58
varicella (chicken pox), 56
yeast infection, 58
iron, 35–36, 43, 38, 104
caffeine and reduced absorption, 46
constipation and, 83
deficiency in, 36, 137, 251
foods high in, 38, 41, 78, 137
for moms of multiples, 255
supplements, 36
itchiness
of breasts, 93
rectal, 85
skin, 29, 80, 92–93
vaginal, 56, 58
when to call your provider, 91

jaundice, 91, 183

Kegel exercises, 65, 83
kick count, 176–77
kidney problems, 19, 225
back pain and, 88
getting pregnant with, 226–27
Klinefelter syndrome, 130

labor
active labor, 170, 171
back labor, 168
back pain as sign of, 88
bleeding and start of, 138
Braxton Hicks contractions, 163
cervix and, 166, 170, 171, 172
childbirth classes to prepare for, 152
contractions, 30, 31, 163–64, 170, 171, 172
contractions, timing, 164
early labor, 170–71
exercise and preparing for, 60, 66
fetal monitoring and, 20
Group B strep and, 57
inducing, 165–67
keeping hydrated, 171
Kegel exercises to prepare for, 65
pain, coping with, 167–69
pain medication, 20, 169
prenatal yoga and, 64
stage 1: contractions, 170–72
stage 2: birth, 172–73
stage 3: afterbirth, 173, 179
transition, 170, 172
La Leche League, 189, 193
lead toxicity, 100–104
lead safety resources, 254
in lipstick, cosmetics, 103, 104
pencils and, 104
room painting and, 105
when to call your provider, 104
leg cramps, 81
when to call your provider, 91
life insurance, 159
lifestyle choices, 16–19
drinking, 17, 233
enlisting support for change, 17
help quitting smoking, drinking, prescription painkillers, or street drugs, 243–44
misusing or abusing prescription narcotic painkillers, 18–19, 234
preconception, 232–36
smoking, 16–17, 233

pain *(continued)*
    in upper-right belly, 90, 141
    when to call your provider, 91, 98, 208
panic attacks, 96, 209
paperwork for pregnancy, 158–59
parvovirus B19 (fifth disease), 57
Patau syndrome (trisomy 13), 125
pediatric provider, 153–54
pelvic exam, 10
perfectionism, 96, 206
perinatologists, 7
perineum, soreness in, 198–99
pertussis, 57
pesticides, 108–11
    avoiding DEET, 109
    dealing with cockroaches, 109–10
pets, 51, 52, 53–54
phenylketonuria (PKU), 48
    maternal, 229–30
phosphorus, 245
physician assistants (PAs), 7–8
pica, 47
placenta, 25, 27
placenta accreta, placenta increta, placenta
        percreta, 264
placental abruption, 138, 149, 263–64
    high blood pressure and, 141, 225
    thrombophilias and, 231
placenta previa, 68, 137–38, 174, 262–63
    limiting activity and, 61
plastics, 112–14
    for baby bottles, 196
    bisphenol A (BPA), 112, 113, 196
    phthalates, 112, 113, 114
    ways to limit your exposure, 113–14
Poison Hotline, 154
polio, 3
postpartum checkup, 210–11
postpartum depression (PPD), 207, 208–10
postpartum psychosis, 210
postpartum symptoms, managing, 206–7
    when to call your provider, 208
post-term pregnancy, 176–77
    testing and, 176–77
Prader-Willi syndrome, 130
preconception, 213–38
    birth control and waiting period, 217
    checkup, 215–16
    chronic medical conditions and, 217–32
    daily multivitamin and, 214, 232
    discussing your health with your pro-
        vider, 216–17

home pregnancy test, 237
lifestyle choices, 232–36
marking your calendar, sex and, 236–37
vaccines, 216
preeclampsia (formerly toxemia), 98, 141,
        142, 222, 225
    HELLP, 141
    thrombophilias and, 231
pregnancy complications, 135–50. *See also*
        specific risk factors
    anemia, 136–37
    avoiding sex and, 68
    bedrest and, 146
    bleeding, 137–38
    cervical insufficiency, 138
    early treatment, 136
    gestational diabetes, 139–40
    high blood pressure, 140–42
    high-risk pregnancies and, 19
    home births and, 21
    hospital nursery classification and, 20
    less common, 260–69
    lowering risk, 15, 16, 59, 135
    MFMs as provider for, 7
    miscarriage, 147–49
    postpartum problems, 200
    prenatal depression, 142–44
    preterm labor and birth, 144–47
    when to call your provider, 91
prenatal care, 6
    answers about workplace chemicals'
        safety, 16
    blood tests, 13–15
    discussion about medications, 11–12
    discussion about multivitamins, 11
    discussion about screening tests, 16
    family's health and genetic history, 13
    first prenatal visit, 9–16
    first-trimester ultrasound, 15
    flu shot, 15
    frequency of appointments, 18
    health and pregnancy history, 12
    importance of appointments, 135
    insurance coverage, 9
    for moms of multiples, 256
    pelvic exam, 10
    physical exam, 10
    picking your provider, 6–9
    plan for managing existing medical con-
        ditions, 13
    planning for delivery of a high-risk baby
        and beyond, 132

urine test, 13
weighing in, 71
when to begin, 6
for women without insurance, 240–41
prenatal depression, 142–44
avoiding herbal remedies, 96
getting help, 257
stress and, 95–96
when to call your provider, 91, 96, 142
prenatal multivitamins, 3, 5, 11, 35, 137, 214
during breastfeeding, 191, 205
following c-section, 202
iron and constipation, 83
iron to prevent anemia and, 14
prenatal testing, 117–33
alternatives to invasive tests, 133
amniocentesis, 123
carrier screening, 119, 121–24
chorionic villus sampling (CVS), 123
diagnostic tests, 119, 124, 127–30
emotional side of, 132–33
for GD, 139–40
screening tests, 119, 124, 125–27
by ultrasound, 125, 131–32
preterm labor and birth, 12, 144–47
bedrest and, 146
care of newborns, 179–80
causes and risk factors, 14, 15, 17, 46,
50, 57, 58, 68, 70, 101, 109, 115, 137,
138, 141 144–45, 231
connecting other parents, 182
exercise and, 61, 62
how to protect yourself, 147
if it happens, 145
lifestyle choices and, 145
March of Dimes research, 4
medicines to prevent, 136
rates in the U.S., 4, 144–47
testing and diagnosis, 146
treatment, 146
what to look for, 88, 145–46
protein, 41–42
breastfeeding and need for, 36
cooking meat, temperatures, 53
good sources, 36, 41–42
how much to have, 42
power bars and energy drinks, 42
recommended intake, 36
why you need it, 41

radon, 108
Rh disease, 14, 149

Rh factor, 14
Rh immune globulin (RhoGAM), 14
riboflavin (vitamin B2), 38
foods high in, 38
rubella (German measles), 14–15, 57, 91
vaccination, 57, 216
rupture of membranes, 164–65
color of fluid, noting, 164

salmonellosis, 51–52
salt, 47, 98
seafood
best choices, 78
DHA and EPA in, 44
fish-eating guidelines, 54
mercury in fish, 44, 54, 106–7, 234–35
pros and cons for pregnant women, 54
seizure disorders
getting pregnant with, 230–31
prenatal care and, 6
sexual activity
avoiding STIs, 55, 68, 234
birth control pills and breastfeeding, 211
during breastfeeding, 192
following c-section, 202
ovulation and conception, 236–37
during pregnancy, 27, 29, 68, 201
resuming after childbirth, 205, 211
sexually transmitted infection (STI), 2, 10
blood tests for, 14
HPV vaccination, 216
recognizing and avoiding, 10, 246
shock, signs of, 208
sickle cell anemia, 130, 224–25
sitz bath, 198, 200
skin
acne, 92
dark spots, 92
facial blood vessels broken, 200
linea nigra, 92
stretch marks, 29, 30, 92
tags, 93
sleep
by baby, 28
back pain and, 88
caring for newborns and, 203–4
leg cramps and, 81
medication, avoiding, 82
mood swings and, 95
mother's need for, 28
mother's positions, 30
naps and, 79, 80

About the Authors

Siobhan Dolan, M.D., M.P.H., is an obstetrician-gynecologist and clinical geneticist who serves as a medical adviser to the March of Dimes. Dr. Dolan is an associate professor in the Department of Obstetrics & Gynecology and Women's Health at the Albert Einstein College of Medicine and an attending physician in the Division of Reproductive Genetics at Montefiore Medical Center, the University Hospital for Einstein, in New York City. She is also on the faculty of the Human Genetics Program at Sarah Lawrence College in Bronxville, New York. Board certified in both OB-GYN and clinical genetics, Dr. Dolan graduated magna cum laude with honors from Brown University and received her medical degree from Harvard Medical School. She did her residency in OB-GYN at the New York Hospital–Cornell Medical Center and Yale–New Haven Hospital and her fellowship in clinical genetics at the Albert Einstein College of Medicine. She received a master's degree in public health from Columbia University.

Dr. Dolan maintains her clinical practice serving women and families in the Bronx. Her research interests focus on the integration of genetics into maternal child health, specifically looking at ways to apply advances in genetics and genomics to improve the health of mothers and babies and prevent birth defects and preterm birth. The mother of three teenagers, she lives with her family in Westchester County, New York.

Alice Lesch Kelly is an award-winning book collaborator and magazine writer specializing in women's health.

She has coauthored seven consumer health books, including *Be Happy Without Being Perfect* and *Conquering Infertility*. Her feature articles have appeared in more than 50 magazines and newspapers, including *Fit Pregnancy, Conceive, Shape, The New York Times, Los Angeles Times, More, Prevention, Good Housekeeping, Health, Parents,* and *O, the Oprah Magazine*. She has been a contributing writer for *Fit Pregnancy* for 10 years. Her work has received awards from the

American Medical Writers Association, the Health Information Resource Center, and the Western Publishing Association.

Kelly earned a bachelor's degree in magazine journalism from Syracuse University and a master's degree in creative writing from Boston University. She teaches nonfiction writing at Emerson College.

She lives in Newton, Massachusetts, with her husband and sons. Her website is www.alicekelly.net.

SCAN THIS CODE

WITH YOUR SMARTPHONE TO BE LINKED TO
THE BONUS MATERIALS FOR

Healthy Mom, Healthy Baby

on the Elixir mobile website,
where you can also find information about other
healthy living books and related materials

YOU CAN ALSO TEXT

MOD to READIT (732348)

to be sent a link to the Elixir mobile website.

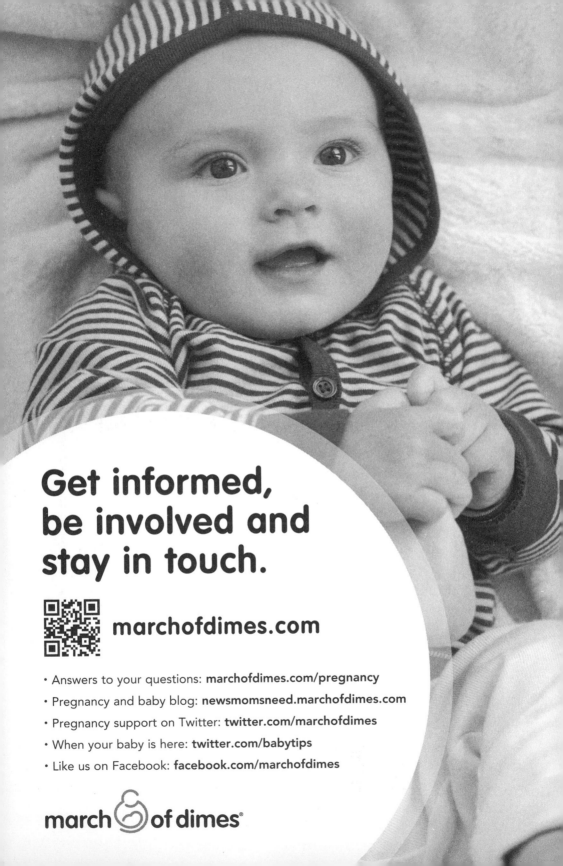

Get informed, be involved and stay in touch.

marchofdimes.com

- Answers to your questions: **marchofdimes.com/pregnancy**
- Pregnancy and baby blog: **newsmomsneed.marchofdimes.com**
- Pregnancy support on Twitter: **twitter.com/marchofdimes**
- When your baby is here: **twitter.com/babytips**
- Like us on Facebook: **facebook.com/marchofdimes**

march of dimes®